face and

FACE AND BODY WAXING COSMETOLOGY

Sub Title

HAIR REMOVAL TRAINING MANUAL

Follows International Standards: - Cosmetology Hair Removal Australian Standards SIBBHRS301A Perform waxing treatments.

Author
Robyna Smith-Keys
Publisher
Robyna Smith-Keys at
Beauty School Books
ISBN: 0994569343
9780994569349
Black and white copy
Also available in full colour
Email **beautyschoolbooks@gmail.com** or robyn@skinsex.com.au
Written August 1999
Revised Version 6 Revised August 2016
Revised May 2021
July 2023

Copyright

Copyright: Naturally you are required to keep the copyright rules.

Copyright Published by

Beauty School Books

Face and Body Waxing - Cosmetology

Table of Contents

Hair Removal Training Manual I

WELCOME TO FACE & BODY WAXING COSMETOLOGY 1

Hair Removal - Training 1

HAIR LENGTH 1

WAX POTS AND ROLLERS 4

HOT WAX POT 4

PROCEDURE - HOT WAX 7

Strip Wax Pot 9

ROLLER WAX 10

Roller wax container 12

Roller Wax Insert 13

ROLLER WAX APLICATION 14

WAXING ROOM EQUIPMENT 18

REMOVING INGROWN HAIRS 20

HOW TO REMOVE INGROWN HAIRS: 21

AROMATHERAPY OBLIGATION 25

Water Based Recipes 28

Alcohol to essential oil ratio 28

- Swing Tags 29
- **AROMATHERAPY EXFOLIATES FOR INGROWN HAIRS.** 31
- **AROMATHERAPY TONER** 32
  - Toner 33
- **AROMATHERAPY CLEANSER** 34
- **EYE MAKEUP REMOVER** 35
- **MOISTURIZER** 37
  - Face MOISTURIZER: - 37
- **AN AGE DEFYING ESSENCE** 39
- **INGROWN HAIR REMOVAL KIT** 41
- **BODY SUGARING** 42
  - How Waxing & Sugaring Works 43
- **SUGAR WAXING** 44
- **SUGAR WAX RECIPE** 45
  - Procedure 45
- **HALAWA SWEET SUGAR WAX** 46
  - Procedure 46
- **FACIAL WAXING** 48
- **LIP & CHIN WAXING** 49

Face and Body Waxing - Cosmetology

CHIN WAXING 52

NOSE HAIR & BLACKHEADS 55

LARGE PORES 56

EAR HAIR 57

    HAIR ON THE EAR LOBES 57

    HAIR INSIDE EARS 58

WOMEN - FACIAL HAIR 58

MEN- BEARDS 59

EYEBROW WAXING 62

EYEBROW ARCH PLACEMENT 66

HAIR THREADING TECHNIQUE 71

    PRACTICE THREADING 73

    BASIC FACTS ON THREADING 74

THREADING DESCRIPTION: 75

    THREADING EYEBROWS ADVANTAGES: 75

    THREADING EYEBROWS DISADVANTAGES: 76

    CLINICAL DATA: 76

    BACKGROUND FACTS 76

GOVERNMENT REGULATION: 77

BASIC BIKINI WAXING STYLES: 78

BIKINI WAX PROCEEDURE 79

    FULL BIKINI WAX: 80

WHEN TO CHOOSE FULL BIKINI WAX 80

FRENCH BIKINI WAX: 81

BRAZILIAN BIKINI WAX: 81

TRIPLE X OR SPHINX 83

NIPPLE WAXING 86

UNDER ARM WAXING 88

    DEEP ARM PIT CHALLENGE. 90

CHEST WAXING WOMEN 90

CHEST WAXING MEN 91

BACK WAXING 95

LEG WAXING 95

KNEE WAXING 97

THIGH - UPPER LEG WAX 98

TOES WAXING 99

OTHER THINGS TO KNOW 102

Face and Body Waxing - Cosmetology

TIPS ON GENITAL AREA WAXING: 104

PRE-BRAZILIAN WAXING PREP: 105

POST BRAZILIAN WAXING CARE: 106

HAIR GROWTH SYSTEM 107

    ANAGEN: 109

    MITOSIS: 109

    CATAGEN: 109

    TELOGEN: 109

HAIR TYPES 110

    LANUGO: 110

    VELLUS: 110

    TERMINAL: 111

    HIRSUTISM: 111

    HYPERTRICHOSIS: 111

    SUPERFLUOUS: 111

HAIR GROWTH 113

BLEACHING 113

    CLIENT RELEASE AND INFORMED CONSENT FOR HAIR BLEACHING/LIGHTENING 114

    HAIR REMOVAL - SHAVING 117

    PHYSICAL HAIR REMOVAL 117

    PHYSICAL HAIR REMOVAL – PLUCKING 118

    PHYSICAL HAIR REMOVAL – WAXING 118

Face and Body Waxing - Cosmetology

AIR BORNE DISEASES 119

QUIZ YOURSELF 120

ABOUT DO'S AND DON'TS 122

DO'S AND DON'TS 123

WAXING PRECAUTIONS & WARNINGS 123

WHEN NOT TO GET WAXED: 126

    WAXING AFTER CANCER TREATMENT 126

WHEN GOLDEN RULES DON'T WORK. 127

DO'S AND DON'TS PHOTO PAGES 128

CLIENTS DO & DON'T HAND OUT 140

ADVICE FOR THE BEAUTY THERAPY INDUSTRY 142

    HEALTH RISKS ASSOCIATED WITH BEAUTY THERAPIES 143
    ULTRAVIOLET LIGHT CABINETS 151
    AUTOCLAVES 152

CLIENT HISTORY CARD 153

OTHER BOOKS BY ROBYNA SMITH-KEYS 158

    HEALING AND TRAINING MANUALS 158
    TRAINING MANUAL- BEAUTY SCHOOLS 158
    YOU MAY CONTACT THE AUTHOR AT 160

FACEBOOK: 160

TWITTER: HTTP://WWW.TWITTER.COM/@AUTHORROBYNA.. 160

MAILTO:BEAUTYSCHOOLBOOKS@GMAIL.COM 160

WELCOME TO FACE & BODY WAXING COSMETOLOGY

HAIR REMOVAL - TRAINING

HAIR LENGTH

Generally, hair needs to be about a centimeter (¼") long for the wax to be able to grab onto. If the hair is not long enough then the hair may not be able to be removed, especially if the hair is thick. But, hair to the other extreme, with too much length, isn't good either.

Waxing Long Hair over a centimeter (2 cm / 1/2" or more) can create other problems.

More breakage. There's more of a chance long hair will break either below or above the skin's surface. Both of these are not good because you'll see the hair faster and you have more of a chance of getting ingrown hair (see: Waxing and Ingrown Hair).

Increased pain. Many people say that it hurts a little bit more if their long, thick hair is removed versus the normal ¼" (read more tips on waxing pain).

Missed hair. When the wax is applied, it pushes hair down flat against the skin. Long hair will cover some of the other hairs. Generally, hair needs to be about 1.5 cm / ¼" long for the wax to be able to grab onto. If it is not long enough then the hair may not be able to be removed, especially if it is thick. But, hair to the other extreme, with too much length, is not good either. Always use the scissor over comb method to shorten hair for easier waxing.

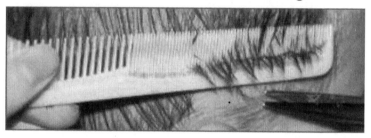

Push comb in the opposite direct to how the hair lays.

The comb is between the skin and the scissors

Place the scissor blade on the comb.

Be sure not to cut too short.

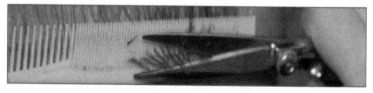

You'll hold the scissors in your dominant hand and cut off hair protruding past the comb, holding the blade parallel to the comb.

Face and Body Waxing - Cosmetology

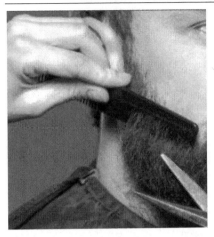

When trimming long hair, ready for the wax procedure do so scissors over comb. Scoop the hair up with the comb, keep the comb firm on the skin and use the scissors to trim the hair. This will prevent you from nicking the clients skin.

You can also electric clippers with the number 2 comb attached.

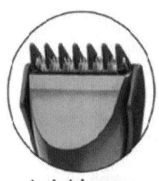

hair trimmer

WAX POTS AND ROLLERS

There are several types of wax and wax methods. Some types of wax, should never be used on the face and we will be discussing all methods and the reasons for each method. There will be your peers, colleges and suppliers that tell you it is fine to use strip wax on the face and I will be telling you it is not acceptable and the reasons why. You will need to read this entire manual then make yourself some notes about the main points.

HOT WAX POT.

Hot wax is used for delicate skin areas. Applied with timber sticks and removed with your fingers.

Hot wax is a very thick wax and is applied thick, then removed with your fingers.

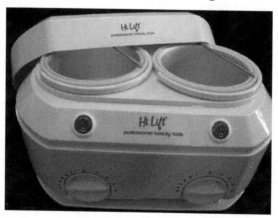

Face and Body Waxing - Cosmetology

Hot wax is usually warmed up in a small thermostat-controlled pot. It is used, for delicate areas such as the face or the vagina plus male and female personal anatomy areas. They come with individual wax pot inserts.

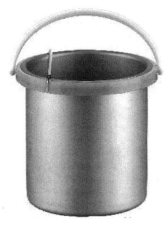

You can heat the wax in the microwave in a microwave safe bowl, then place in the metal pot in the wax warmer. Alternately, you can turn the heat control button onto high for 10 minutes. Set a timer so you do not forget to turn the heat control button back down to "1" after ten minutes. You may leave the pot on heat number 1 all day if you're in a Salon. The wax must be warm enough to penetrate the hair. Yet not so hot that it is runny.

Be sure to check the wax throughout the day and turn it off at night before you leave the Salon.

Note: For home users if you cannot afford a waxing pot like this you can simply purchase the metal pot inserts and put the wax in the pot in a fry pan. Fill the pan with boiling water do not have the water too high up the side of the wax pot and keep the water simmering not boiling. When the wax has reached the desired temperature, take it out of the fry pan and start waxing. As the wax cools down return, it to the fry pan. You can also use a double sauce pan.

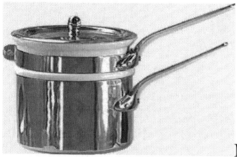

May I suggest, you do not use this pot for anything else.

PROCEDURE - HOT WAX

Naturally, it will depend on the body part to be waxed, but this is the general rule.

- Do your meet and greet, with the client and fill in his / her client forms.
- Take his / her to the waxing room and explain where they can put their belongings such as clothes, shoes bag and so on.
- If they are wearing jewellery, have them wrap it in a tissue and place in their shoes. That way they are sure to put their jewellery back on when the treatment has been, completed. If they put it in their pocket or bag, they may forget about it. They could misplace their jewellery on the way home and think they have left it at the Salon. Be firm about this. It is your good name, you are protecting.
- Explain where you want the client to sit or lay.
- Leave them to get ready.
- Check hair length.
- Trim long hairs to 1.5 cm (1/4")
- Apply skin cleaner
- Apply a prep oil or talc (ask manufacturers what they Recommend)

- Apply hot wax thickly with timber sticks Never re-dip the stick into the pot.
- Press into the skin
- Remove with fingers
- Press the area with your palm
- Repeat steps 3, 4 and 5 until area has been completed.
- Excess wax can be removed with wax. Put a small amount on your finger and press onto the extra wax and hold skin firm and remove in a rolling motion.
- Place a cold wet cloth on the waxed area. (This is a very important step do not skip this step.)
- Clean skin with oil. Put oil in one hand rub your hands together. Now run your well-oiled hands over the waxed skin firmly. Do not allow your fingers to press into the skin, tilt your fingers upward as you use your palms to remove wax.
- Tissue off excess.
- Apply after wax solution.

STRIP WAX POT

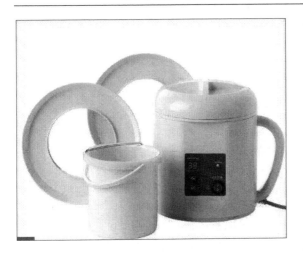

Strip Wax is usually heated in a larger pot. Applied with a wooded spatula and removed with strips of cloth.

Strip wax is a runny yet thick type of wax. When cold it is dark in colour. When heated it is usually transparent. To learn the correct consistency and heat for waxing takes time and practice. Always test on yourself for heat before placing on a client. **WARNING.** If too hot it will remove skin and flesh.

ROLLER WAX

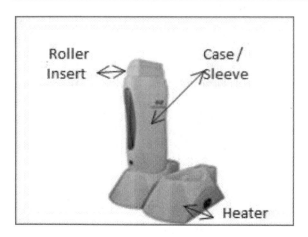

Roller waxes are known as strip wax. The method is the same as for strip wax. The difference is at the top of the pot of wax cartilage there is a roller that you roll over the skin.

The plastic cartilage/pot sits in a thermostat-controlled heater.

You must roll the wax onto cloth to see if it is at the right temperature and consistency.

It should spread like warm honey.

When you apply to the skin, hold the roller pot at 45-degree angle to the skin. Never hold and drag on the skin at right angles to the skin. It must be applied as a thin layer.

You will use cloth strips to remove the wax. Never ever, attempt to roll over long hair.

For leg waxing, roller waxing is by far my favorite, but never ever use on long hair. You should trim long hair first.

Roller wax method is for body waxing only not the face. Suppliers do make small rollers for eyebrows and upper lips but, there are several reasons why you should **not** buy and use these units.

1. It is not cost effective to buy the small roller inserts for lips and eyebrows.

2. Each insert is for a single use. You cannot under Australian Health and Safety Regulations use the same roller on more than one client.

3. The Roller and the wax container are attached. The roller is plastic and cannot be sterilized before using on the next client.

Rollers pull the skin therefore the roller style wax is unsuitable for facial waxing.

Some suppliers offer rollers for the lip and eyebrows. They give an unprofessional finish to the job.

ROLLER WAX CONTAINER

Roller wax heaters come in single or multiple

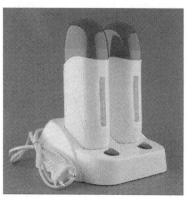

stands. Most types of wax pots and rollers have a temperature control button. See manufactures instructions. Note how this heater has a white sleeve. This is the best kind of heater unit. The wax is hot to hold and when the heater does not have a sleeve for the wax to sit in you have to put a cloth around the wax insertion unit so you do not burn your hand while rolling the wax on the skin.

> Note: This double roller unit has a charging base. You can purchase these in a single unit as well. What is great about this unit type is: you take the cap off the top and the wax sits inside the case. This means you do not remove the wax container.

Some units have the power attached to the case and they do not have a charging unit. They are a bothersome because as you remove the roller from the case, you need to put a cloth around the wax cartridge.

ROLLER WAX INSERT.

Roller wax insertions (cartridge) come pre-packaged.

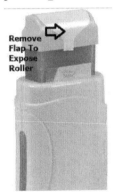

The wax is in a container and the container has a roller unit attached. Some heaters have a stand that you place this unit into. Then you remove this unit and wrap it in cloth while you roll the wax onto the skin.

As per the above photo, it is best to buy a heating unit with a sleeve that the wax cartridge slots into. Then you remove the cartridge which stays inside the container, while you roll the wax onto the skin.

Note: The rollers cannot be sterilized. Therefore, you cannot use this wax roller on another client.

> 2nd Note: Always roll the wax onto a strip of cloth before rolling onto the client. This will get the roller moving freely and assist you to visualize the consistence.

> 3rd Note: Hold the wax roller at 45 degrees to the skin as you roll. Be sure to do so with pressure. You are trying to push the wax through the skin and into the pours of the skin.

ROLLER WAX APLICATION

Notice how this Therapist is <u>pulling the skin</u> as she rolls at 45 degrees to the skin. Rolling in the direction of the hair growth and she is stretching the skin by pulling down on the skin, the way the hair would lay on the skin. That works fine but. I prefer you to cup your hand around the top of the leg above where you are waxing and pull the skin in the opposite direction to the way you are applying the wax.

It is also advisable to have the client bend their knee with their foot flat on the bed as per the second photo.

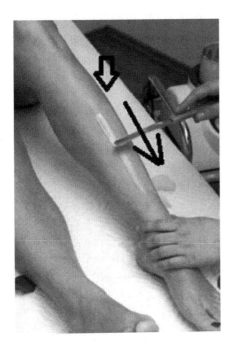

Note The Leg Should Be Bent And The Toes Pointed. When they point their toes it creates tighter skin and hurts less.

- When the client is asked to point their toes this helps by

- Making the skin firm and their fore hurts less as you remove the wax.
- Strip Wax Procedure

1. Prepare Client. Do your meet and greet and fill in her / his client forms.
2. Take him or her to the waxing room and explain where they can put their belongings such as clothes, shoes, bag and so on.
3. If they are wearing jewellery, have them wrap it in a tissue and place in their shoes. That way they are sure to put their jewellery back on when the treatment is completed. If they put it in their pocket or bag, they may forget about it. They could lose the jewellery on the way home and think they have left it at the Salon. Be firm about this. It is your good name, you are protecting.
4. Explain where you want the client to sit or lay.
5. Leave them to get ready.
6. Trim hair that is more than 1cm in length.
7. Apply skin cleaner.
8. Apply a prep oil or talc (ask wax manufacturers what they recommend as

each manufacturers wax has their own method.)

9. Apply wax thickly with timber sticks. Never re-dip the stick into the pot. You can however, use the other end of the stick. Once you have applied the wax to the skin wrap a tissue around the waxy end.

10. Remove the wax then you can hold the tissue covered end of the wax stick and dip the other end of the stick into the pot.

11. Spread onto the skin very thinly

12. Remove with strips of calico, linen, or denim. When you place the denim/calico/linen strip onto the waxed area, rub the cloth with the palm of your hand, applying some friction.

13. Hold the skin at the top of the cloth and pull the skin to stretch the skin as you pull the cloth and wax off.

14. When you remove wax, do so in a fast swift motion. Do so in the direction opposite to hair growth and parallel to the skin.

15. Press your hand onto the area to remove pain.

16. Repeat until area has been completed.

17. Clean skin with astringent then oil.

18. Apply after wax solution suitable for the area being waxed.

19. I like to apply a cold cloth for a few minutes, then the after-wax oil.

20. Show your professionalism and give the clients above average care. They are your best form of advertising.

WAXING ROOM EQUIPMENT

- A Metal Trolley
- Refrigerator, with freezer section.
- Ice Packs
- Heat Bags
- Basin with hot and cold running water
- Hot wax
- Strip wax
- Hot wax pot
- Strip wax pot
- Roller wax and stand (optional)
- Cardboard rings for your pots.
- Cotton for Threading
- Cotton strips
- Denim strips
- Linen strips
- Eye Pads
- Head bands

- Metal spatula for stirring wax
- Paddle pop sticks
- Tongue depressors.
- Gentle exfoliate brushes made from coconut shell.
- Talcum powder
- Cleanser
- Toner
- Prep oil
- After wax oil
- Before wax oil
- Before wax astringent
- Cotton swabs
- Cotton balls
- Cotton wool squares/rounds
- Tweezers made for ingrown hairs
- Eyebrow tweezers
- Scissors
- Bikini stencils
- Alcohol
- Hydrogen peroxide
- Paper Towels
- Tissues
- Paper bed roll
- Gloves
- Oil dissolver
- Eucalyptus oil
- Lavender oil
- Olive oil
- Coconut oil

- Calipers
- Eyebrow stencils
- Eyebrow powder
- Eyebrow pencils.
- Aftercare products to sell to clients.

- White face cloths. (As they can be bleached or boiled for purification)

REMOVING INGROWN HAIRS

Removing ingrown hairs isn't exactly hard but does require prepping the skin and the right post care for the best possible results. Every client is different and has a different type of hair structure. Some ladies may have hairs on their body parts as strong as a thick black beard of a male. Naturally, their ingrown hair problem will be harder to cure - than a fair skin person with natural blonde hair. Also, those who eat lots of fresh raw fruit and vegetables usually have a quicker healing rate.

If the hair is infected or severely inflamed, physically removing the hair can irritate the skin further because it's in a fragile state, so please use precaution. Explain to the client why you cannot remove the hair and what her before and aftercare options are. You will need to also explain why you cannot wax someone with infected ingrown hairs.

How you explain that to a client without offending them takes mindful skills. For most of you studying body waxing - you would have already learnt about "Air Borne Diseases" when you did your Beauty Diploma.

Therefore, it is not my intension in this manual to go through what you should already know. If you are a Hairdresser wanting to add waxing services to your business, may I suggest you do the skin penetration module. I have added a brief section on Air Borne Diseases below.

HOW TO REMOVE INGROWN HAIRS:

Consider this as an after-care sheet that you make up to give the client.

Put Your Salon Name and Telephone number at the head of the page and reduce the size of the print so it fits on one page.

Naturally, a twenty-minute swim in a clean River or the Ocean 3-5 times a week cures almost any skin sores.

Should the Ocean be nearby, make good use of the healing powers and swim., often.

Develop a daily habit of drinking freshly made fruit and vegetable juices.

1. **Cleanse skin.** Use a mild cleanser to rid skin of surface dirt and debris.

2. **Apply heat.** Take a warm shower or bath or apply a very warm washcloth over the infected area for about five minutes.

3. The heat helps to soften skin, relax the hair follicle, and aid hair in coming to the surface.

4. **Exfoliate area.** Using a mild exfoliate, use fingertips in small circles around hair follicle to loosen debris and dead skin, then rinse. If you do not have a mild exfoliate use 1 tablespoon of Olive oil and a pinch of salt. Mix the oil and salt together in a small bowl. Throw away the left-over mix and use a fresh mix again within a few days. Less is best with the salt. Too much salt will aggravate the inflamed skin around the follicle. You may also use a pitch of bicarbonate of soda.

5. Warm Cloth. Again, press a warm wet facecloth to the area. Use the cloth one

6. time only and soak in nappy sanitizer or water, detergent, and bleach. You can use a large pierce of cotton wool soaked in warn water and put the facecloth over the cotton wool.

7. **Remove hair.** Try to gently remove hair by holding skin taut, and 'scraping' a cotton swab over the ingrown hair, in the opposite direction of the ingrown hair. If the hair comes out, then skip the next step.

8. **Try tweezers.** Use tweezers especially made for ingrown hairs with a rounded tip. Ingrown hair tweezers, must first be sanitize with alcohol. Gently grab onto hair and only remove the hair growing into the skin, but don't take hair out from root because this will irritate the hair follicle further.

9. **Shave hair.** Once ingrown hair is out of the skin, then shave it down if it's much longer than surrounding hair with a clean blade and shaving cream or gel. You should charge the client for this extra service or have an aftercare leaflet make up so she/he can perform this duty at home.

10. **Disinfect area.** Apply a small amount of 10 volume hydrogen peroxide with

11. a clean cotton ball or gauge square to hair follicle and then Neosporin to ward off infection. 10 volume means that 10% of the liquid is peroxide and 90% is distilled water. Or 10 ml of peroxide and 90 ml of water.
I prefer to clean and tone the area with Aromatherapy cleanser and toner. See notes in Aromatherapy section.

You can make this ingrown hair product and name it here. Be sure to have stock available for the client to purchase.

12. **Break them off.** While this works well for an ingrown here and there, that's really bothering your client, using a product specifically for ingrown hair. A serum made for this challenge can help remove ingrown hairs or avoid them altogether.

13. Also, see my tips for products you can make. Again, I would prefer you to offer the clients Aromatherapy products that you make.

Tips:
1. Don't dig tweezers or scissors hard into skin and leave a mark.
2. Be sure the skin is warm and the ingrown hair tweezers and scissors have been sterilized.
3. Hold the skin as if you were trying to pull the pour open.

Now make the before and after leaflet to give to clients. You should not charge them for this leaflet.

AROMATHERAPY OBLIGATION

It is your obligation to look at a recipe and adjust it to the blending safety and precaution rules.

Not all recipes are written with all the safety measures.
1. Essential Oils cannot be safely applied to the skin neat.
2. Essential oils do not blend with water.

Face and Body Waxing - Cosmetology

3.

Carrier	Essential Oil For Body 2%	Carrier	Essential Oil For Face 1%
100 ml	50 drops	100 ml	25 drops
50 ml	25 drops	50 ml	12 to 13 drops
25 ml	12 to 13 drops	25 ml	10 drops
20 ml	10 drops	20 ml	5 drops
10 ml	5 drops	10 ml	2 drops
5 ml	2 drops	5 ml	1 drop

This chart is available on ebay.com.au or on https://beautyschoolbooks.com.au/safety-chart/

There are also some free instructions

Essential Oils.

Essential oil dilution is important for two safety reasons. One, to avoid skin reactions: irritation, sensitization and phototoxicity. Two, to avoid systemic toxicity, such as fetotoxicity, hepatotoxicity, carcinogenicity, and neurotoxicity. Adverse skin reactions are obvious when they happen, but systemic toxicities may not be. Skin reactions are totally dilution-dependent, and safety guidelines exist to minimize risk.

WATER BASED RECIPES

Water in any product needs to be considered the enemy. Water used in the formulation of cosmetics is not your everyday, regular tap water. It must be 'ultra-pure'—that is, free from microbes, toxins, and other pollutants. For this reason, your label may refer to it as distilled water, purified water or just aqua.

When a recipe calls for water, you need to use distilled water.

When adding essential oils to a water-based product - you must first render the essential oils miscible, before adding to the water.

At proper concentration, ethanol/95% Alcohol "marries" essential oils and water together, so they become one homogeneous substance that can no longer be separated into two distinct substances. There can be no separation or 'divorce', they're forced to stay together for good! Consider high proof "Everclear" as your alcohol of choice until you learn more.

ALCOHOL TO ESSENTIAL OIL RATIO

The ratio is 1 in 4. 1 drop of essential oil to 4 drops of alcohol. This is the safest way to blend essential oils when adding them to a water-based recipe. If the recipe fails to tell you this you now know what to do.

SWING TAGS

Aromatherapy products that you can make in the salon will need a swing tag with the ingredients listed. I make tags that fold in half. I type the information and stick on black or purple cards. I cover the card with wide sticky tape so it lasts longer.

You could also laminate the card.

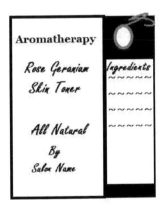

You can buy blue aromatherapy bottles from the Bottle People or New Directions or buy secondhand bottles. Sterilize them and decorate them.

All bottles and jars must be a dark glass or food safe plastic.

If the jars and bottles are clear glass that you are recycling or have purchased to make gift oils they need to be thoroughly cleaned and the outside must be painted or decorated so no natural light gets into the bottle.

Light destroys the healing properties of essential oils as they are volatile liquids.
http://www.pbpackaging.com.au/
http://www.newdirections.com.au/
New Directions also sell essential oils.

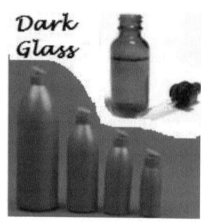

AROMATHERAPY EXFOLIATES FOR INGROWN HAIRS.

Place 100 ml Olive oil in a dark-coloured narrow neck bottle add: -

10 drops of rose geranium and 10 drops of lemon essential oil 5 drops Frankincense.

You can make this oil and sell to your client with the below instructions.

Shake and keep in a cool dark place.

Grind some sea salt and pepper together and place in a small glass jar or PTFE plastic Jar.

Add half a teaspoon of the salt and pepper mix to 3 tablespoons of the oil blend

Exfoliate the skin in a circular motion with this mix. Do this every night the first week, then twice a week for one more week, then once a week thereafter.

After the exfoliating, rinse off with warm water, pat dry with cotton wool and wipe with a cotton pad soaked in toner. Then take a warm not hot shower.

Should you not like nor have the time for this incredibly wonderful oil exfoliate, you can help stop ingrown hairs with a beauty brush.

The best exfoliate brush to use is one made from coconut shell. Spend five minutes twice a week circulating the brush over the skin before a warm oil bath or shower.

After a shower, you will need to massage in the above oil blend. Be sure to rinse off with warm soapy water.

Before bed place a little toner onto the skin and wipe off with cotton wool pads.

AROMATHERAPY TONER

Before you begin making toner read Water in Oil Advise.

You can just use watered down apple cider vinegar or this wonderful mix: -

In a clean dark bottle with a spray top add

30% witch hazel and 60% boiled water that has been allowed to cool down.

In 5ml 95% alcohol Add 10 drops of rose geranium, 3 drops Clary sage and 3 drops of Eucalyptus or Lemon essential oils. Shake and use. However, the essential oils will need to be made miscible with alcohol before adding to the mix. The alcohol needs to be 95% or 115 proof.

TONER

In a 100 ml dark coloured narrow neck bottle place 85 ml of cooled boiled water. Preferably use distilled water.

Add 10 ml witch hazel
10 drops of Essential oil.
5 Drops Rose Geranium,
5 Drop Clary Sage
2 Drop Eucalyptus **or** Frankincense
Use above ratio to make the essential oils miscible in alcohol then add to the blend. Shake well.

Frankincense is a natural skin toner that reduces pores but is very expensive and is a very strong sedative that can stupefy the brain if over used.

If you have acne add one drop only of Tea tree Essential oil, and 3 drops Ylang Ylang in place of Clary Sage.

Ylang Ylang essential oil has a rich, floral fragrance. It helps to control oil production and minimize breakouts. It also helps regenerate skin cells, smoothing fine lines and improving skin elasticity. A great essential oil, for every skin type.

Tea tree oil is widely advertised as being a good healer for acne and pus related skin disorders. However, I have experienced the drying out of healthy skin cells and I am not a lover of tea tree oil.

AROMATHERAPY CLEANSER

Place 95 to 100 milligrams (3.3 Ounces} of cold pressed olive or grape-seed oil into a 100 ml dark coloured narrow neck bottle.

Add 5-10 drops of your chosen Essential oils. Shake and you're done.

Note: This cleanser can also double as a massage blend and a moisturizer.

Be sure to add a pump as the cap so you do not need to add a preservative. Give the label a six months shelf life to protect yourself.

It is important after you or your client tissues off the cleanser to complete the cleaning process with a warm wet face cloth. Press into the skin repeat as you wipe the skin with a fresh warm wet face cloth.

EYE MAKEUP REMOVER

Eye makeup remover, for stubborn eye makeup.
Place in a small dark clean glass bottle.
50 ml Olive oil or baby oil
10 Drops of Chamomile Essential oil.
Never use baby oil for massage blends.
You can also use coconut oil. Either straight, from the jar or place 10 tablespoons of coconut oil in a clean dark jar and add 5 drops of chamomile essential oils. Other essential oils that are good for the eye area are: -

Rose
Clary sage
Rose geranium
However whenever possible use Chamomile as the preferred oil.

For after care Almond or Jojoba oils are great especially if you add either the essential oils of chamomile, rose geranium or rose otto.

- With your fingertips gently massage a few drops onto a closed eye. Do one eye at a time. Stay within the eye area and do not massage for more than a few seconds.

- Also, do not spread the oil too far away from the eye area as you are dissolving eye makeup. You do not want to push eye makeup into the skin. You want to dilute it.

- Remove with cotton wool pads.

- Then sponge off with a warm wet face cloth.

- Pat the skin dry.

- Gentle wipe closed eyes over with cotton wool soaked in water and toner. By using a wet cotton wool pad, the toner will be diluted.

When you wet the cotton, pad squeeze out excess water then spay with toner.

Note: If using coconut oil, you will need to place into a jar not a bottle as it sets hard. **Warning.** This is for the external eyelid not to be put onto the actual eye.

Read this report.
http://roberttisserand.com/2013/02/essential-oils-and-eye-safety/

MOISTURIZER

Moisturizer is simple to make. Use 100 ml of base oils such as Jojoba or greased oil.

Add 10 drops of essential oils. Gently massage onto your skin twenty minutes before applying makeup. Also, tone the skin before applying the moisturizer and again before applying makeup.

FACE MOISTURIZER: -

This is my favorite face moisturizer as it can be massages close to the eyes.
 In a clean dark glass bottle
Place 100 ml of Jojoba oil
add: -
3 Drops of Rose Essential oil
 2 Drops of Clarysage
10 Drops of Ylang Ylang.

I actually prefer Olive oil and Coconut oil as my base oil, for a moisturizer. In my, daily skincare routine, I never use moisturizer during the day.

Your body is pulsating outwards and actually is irritated by moisturizers.

Rose oil has over 500 healing properties but is very expensive. Rose Geranium works profoundly on the emotions, acne, bruises, burns, cuts, dermatitis, eczema, hemorrhoids, lice, mosquito repellent, ringworm, ulcers, edema, poor circulation, sore throat, tonsillitis, PMS, menopausal problems, stress, and neuralgia. Rose Geranium does not have all the healing properties of Rose oil but is a good substitute when you cannot afford Rose oil.

Rose (Rosa Damascena) essential oil is one of the most expensive. Rose oil is difficult to extract; it takes several thousand rose petals to produce a minute quantity of oil.

Geranium (Pelargonium graveolens) essential oil is an acceptable substitute for rose oil. Although rose oil and geranium oil are made up of different chemical components, in different quantities, they both contain a high content of alcohols. In addition, both of these essential oils are popular with women and are used for many skincare complaints.

It can also be used to remedy digestive ailments, kidney and bladder disorders and has traditionally been considered as an astringent. As well as keeps ticks away from animals.

Clary Sage is reputed to contain phytohormones with estrogen-like properties it is favored as an 'anti-aging' factor in skin care preparations.

AN AGE DEFYING ESSENCE

It is good for puffiness of the skin and fluid retention with tonic and soothing properties.

Body Moisturizer - All Skin Types
In a dark clean glass bottle add: -
In 100 ml of olive oil
Add 10 drops Clary Sage or Rose Geranium.
Add 10 Drops Ylang Ylang

Olive oil can easily be replaced with coconut oil. However, as the coconut oil is much thicker place it in a jar. The healing properties are almost the same with either the olive or the coconut oil. The coconut oil will work quicker at moisturizing very dry skin, Olive oil is by far my favourite in a healing blend. Fractionated coconut is a better liquid form of coconut but does not have the same benefits. Placing oils or creams in a jar calls for a preservative.

INGROWN HAIR REMOVAL KIT

- A gentle exfoliates (as per above mix) or purchase one.
- Warm Water
- Towels
- Face Cloths
- Ingrown Hair Tweezers
- Scissors with rounded point
- Cleanser
- Toner
- Aromatherapy massage oil
- Cotton swabs
- Alcohol to sterilize tools
- Cotton balls or squares

BODY SUGARING

Body sugaring is a must learn, for the modern Wax Therapist.

Summer means overtime in the hair removal department and dollars in your till.

Master this ancient art of body sugaring. Apparently, this is how Cleopatra and her group kept their legs enchantingly smooth, and thoroughly modern misses have recently started buzzing about it too.

Sugaring works a lot like waxing - a paste is smothered over hair-baring areas, and then whipped off with cloth strips - only with two major plus points.

A sugar-based wax sticks only to hair, the theory being that this will not sting the skin when stripped off.

Made from gentle, natural ingredients and applied at room temperature, it gives sensitive skin a relief.

HOW WAXING & SUGARING WORKS

Waxing is the application of a sticky substance to skin. The resin binds hair to a strip of cloth, which is pulled off (always in the opposite direction of hair growth). Hair is removed, from the roots and will eventually grow back. However, not all hair will grow back. Some of the wax will penetrate the sebaceous gland and the hair root will also be removed. This is fine in most areas but on the eyebrows, this can be devastating.

Sugaring, an alternative to wax, is made up of a mixture of lemon juice, sugar, and water. Hair needs to be at least 1 cm long for the waxing to work. Because - the wax needs to bind on the hair in order for it to be yanked out. The pain factor here is moderate to high and more so during your menstruation period. The first time hurts the most. Hair grows back thinner. After a couple times it hurts a bit less. Waxing and sugaring, lasts about 2 to 6 weeks.

SUGAR WAXING

Sugar waxing is a popular form of hair removal that works in the same way traditional waxing does. A thick sugary substance similar to caramel is spread on the skin in the direction of hair growth. The hair becomes, embedded, in the caramel. A cloth or paper strip, is patted onto the caramel and then pulled off quickly, in the opposite direction, of the hair growth, pulling the hairs out of the follicles. The advantage of this method over traditional waxing is the clean-up. The sugar substance is water-soluble and can be removed easier than wax by rinsing with water.

Once you become at sugar waxing there will be no need to use cloth to remove the wax from the skin. You roll onto the skin and roll off with your fingers.

SUGAR WAX RECIPE

2 cups of sugar,
1/4 cup of lemon juice
1/4 cup of water,
2 drops of Chamomile Essential Oil

Add essential oil to 8 drops of 95% alcohol. Not vodka.

PROCEDURE

Mix and heat all ingredients except the Chamomile oil until the blend looks caramel-like, then let it stand until almost cool. This is when you stir in the Chamomile alcohol mix. Place in a jar until it's pliable and cool enough to slather on with a spatula. Make a large batch and store in small foil pie cups until ready to use. As soon as this mix is made boil the kettle and put the boiling water in the pan then rinse it in an unused part of your garden. I pour it on a thick layer of newspaper then when cool and hard I throw it in the garbage. Keep the pot full of water until you scrub it clean. Do not use this pot for any other purpose and be sure it is a heavy based pot made of stainless steel. Never use an aluminum pot.

Try this at home several times before trying it on clients. Once you get it right you will have very happy clients.

It leaves the skin feeling very silky and it does not take skin with it when you use it.

Now days you can buy rubber cake tins buy a few muffins sized, rubber baking dishes and store the extra wax in them. These types of pans can be placed into the microwave to preheat the wax.

HALAWA SWEET SUGAR WAX

1. Two cups of water
2. Three cups of sugar or three cups of honey
3. Two teaspoons of lemon juice

PROCEDURE

Place all ingredients in saucepan. Bring to boil.

When its colour changes to golden brown, lower the heat and continue to simmer. Keep a careful watch on the colour. Once it starts to change to brown, turn off the heat.

LIP & CHIN WAXING

- Meet and greet and fill in the client history card.
- Warm the lip/chin with a warm wet face cloth. I use a tiny heat bag that I heat the bag in the microwave for 40 seconds. I wrap it in paper tow and place on the clients lip for one minute.

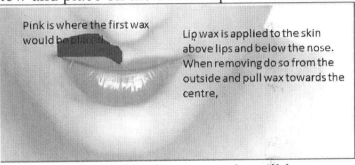

Pink is where the first wax would be placed.

Lip wax is applied to the skin above lips and below the nose. When removing do so from the outside and pull wax towards the centre,

Clean the area with cleanser and a mild toner.
- Apply pre-wax oil wipe off excess with cotton wool
- Put the hot wax on one side of the top lip with a large amount of wax on the **outside** of the lip. Like a tab.
- Press the wax into the skin.
- Place a small amount or hot wax on your thumb and press into the outside lump of wax on the lip.
- Use one hand to pull the skin in the opposite direction to the way you will pull the wax off.

- With pointy finger and thumb, remove the wax.
- Press your palm firmly on the lip for 20 seconds. This is a very important step as it calms the nerves under the skin.
- Repeat steps 4-10 on the other side of the lip.
- Repeat for the center of the lip. However, you pull upwards towards the nose when removing the wax.
- When you have completed the left side of the lip. Place the palm of your hand over the entire lip area.
- Place a cold wet face cloth immediately on the lip for two minutes.
- Repeat above steps for the right side of the lip.
- Place a very gentle toner on a cotton wool pad, pat the lip.
- Apply Jojoba oil on the lip or moisturizer.
- Be certain to start the wax removal at the outer side of the lips.
- Treat the outer corner of the lips separately.
- Ask the client to smile with her mouth closed.
- Always complete the wax with an ice pack or piece of ice.

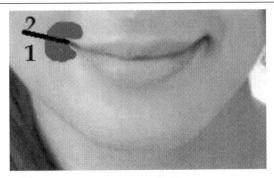

Apply the wax in two sections and remove a section before applying the next section of wax.

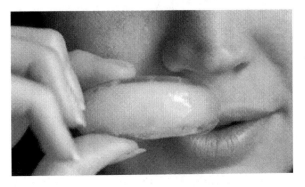

Always finish with an ice pack.

CHIN WAXING

After your meet and greet and filling in the client

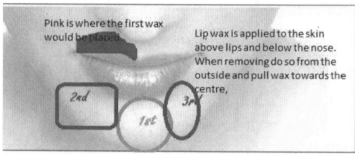

card.

- Clean the area with cleanser and toner.
- Warm the chin with a warm wet face cloth. I use a tiny heat bag that I heat in the microwave for 40 seconds. I wrap it in paper towel Test the heat on my wrist and place on the clients chin for one minute.
- Apply pre-wax oil
- Put the hot wax on one side of the upper chin area, with a large amount of wax on the outside of the chin. Like a tab.
- Press the wax into the skin.
- Place a small amount or hot wax on your thumb and press into the outside lump of wax on the chin.

- Use one hand to pull the skin in the opposite direction to the way you will pull the wax off.
- With your pointy finger and thumb remove the wax.
- Press you palm firmly on the chin for 20 seconds. This is a very important step as it calms the nerves under the skin.
- Repeat steps 4-10 on the other side of the chin.
- Repeat for the center of the chin however, you pull upwards towards the nose when removing the wax.
- For under the chin. Repeat above instructions in sections.
- Place the palms of your hands over the entire chin area.
- Place a cold wet face cloth immediately on the chin for two minutes.
- Place a very gentle toner on a cotton wool pad and pat the chin.
- Apply Jojoba oil on the chin.

1. The chin is almost as sensitive as the lip, so be sure to follow these instructions.
2. Keep the skin well pulled while removing the wax.

3. Place your palm firmly on the skin immediately as you remove each section of wax.

4. Be sure to use the hot and cold cloths.

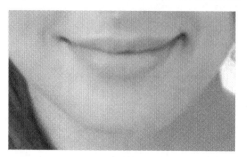

5. For both lip and chin waxing you should ask the client to create a broad/wide closed mouth smile. This will assist you and the client to keep the skin stretched tight.

NOSE HAIR & BLACKHEADS

Nose waxing is not just about removing hair from the nose. Placing wax on the top tip of the nose and pressing it into the pores removes white and blackheads better than any other blackhead remover.

For many years they have been selling nose pads with a cold wax on them or sticky nose pads for removing blackheads. Why they do not teach you this blackhead removal technique in beauty schools today is beyond me.

Treat the nose the same way you would the chin and use the same method to remove blackheads and hairs from the outside of the nose. Only use hot wax not strip waxes.

1. For internal hair in the nose clean the nose out with tissues and toner.
2. Have the client blow their nose into a tissue before you begin.
3. Put some wax on your pointy finger press it into the inside of the nose.
4. Keep your finger there with pressure.
5. Use a rocking method and have your thumb join your other finger and pull out the wax.

6. Be sure to stretch the nose skin with the other hand.

Only remove hairs close to the nose hole do not go deep into the nose. Unless the client is blind, they should trim their inner nose hair themselves.

LARGE PORES

Waxing the skin can help reduce the pore size. Black heads increase the size of your pores. When you cleanse the skin, use a mild toner to complete the cleaning process. You will find the pore size will reduce. Place wax on the outside of the nose in small sections. Remove the section before applying wax to the next section.

Some people are born with larger than normal skin pores. These large pores can largely be attributed to their genetic makeup.

Certain areas of body such as nose, forehead and central area of the face generally tend of have bigger pores for both, men and women secreting more sebum (body oil). At times, these openings become jammed with dirt and dead skin cells leading to formation of blackheads and whiteheads and therefore making these openings appear even larger.

Unfortunately, there is no magic wand which can shrink these pores to the preferred size and make their skin appear younger and vibrant. However, waxing and toning will help. These people need to cleanse, exfoliate and tone more religiously than people with small pores.

Retin-A and salicylic acid helps to reduce oil production in the glands and skin exfoliation. Caution! When using this treatment always consult a medical professional.

The amount and frequency of the dosage is absolutely critical and can be very harmful to your health if proper precautions are not followed.

Aromatherapy products are safer.
See My Book Called " Natural Organic Skincare Recipes" for more skin repair recipes.

EAR HAIR

HAIR ON THE EAR LOBES

Long hairs will need to be trimmed first. Hair on the lobes of the ears is very tough and well rooted. Use the same method as you would for the chin. Be sure to pull the lobe down towards the shoulders, firmly as you remove the hot wax. Never ever, use a strip wax on the ears.

HAIR INSIDE EARS

Do not attempt to remove hairs from the inside of the ear with wax. If you trim the hairs, put cotton wool in the ears. Add one eye drop of Olive oil to the cotton wool then use sterilized surgical steel scissors to trim the hair. Remove the cotton wool carefully so the hairs do not fall back into the ear.

Place a drop of toner on a cotton pad and wipe the inside of the ear out.

WOMEN - FACIAL HAIR

Some women have facial hairs that are blonde and show up more when they apply makeup. The pronounced hairs are usually around the outer cheek areas. It is my recommendation that we teach them how to apply a foundation in such a way that the hairs do not show up as much and encourage then to have a hair style that comes onto the face. A wispy hair style that flicks on to the face is better than them having the facial hairs waxed.

Should they be unwavering, about having the hair removed use the hot wax method.

- Do your meet and greet.
- Fill in client forms
- Cleanse and tone the skin

Face and Body Waxing - Cosmetology

- Apply pre-wax oil
- Apply hot wax
- Remove with your fingers
- Apply a mild toner to the skin
- Then apply Jojoba oil.

If hair is strong or thick use a warm compress before the waxing and after the cleaning process.

MEN- BEARDS

The question is - should you or should you not wax a mans beard. Well, that depends on these things: -

- How tough is his beard and how strong is the hair in his beard?
- Is he prepared for the pain?
- Is he a trim or plump man?
- If his is suitable, is he happy to have part of his bead waxed and shave the rest of his face.
- If so, is he happy to slowly build up to a full facial wax?
- Does he drink alcohol each night after work?

- Is he taking medication or drugs?

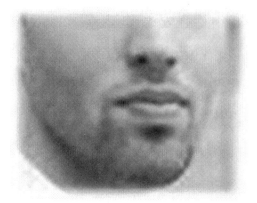

-
- This man beard is too tough for waxing even though he is a slim build and has no flabby skin.

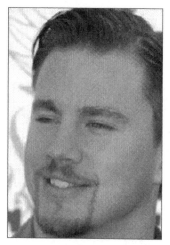

- This man has a different kind of hair on his upper lip to the hair on his face. Therefore, he could have some of his face waxed. The hair on his chin is stronger type of hair and should not, be waxed.

- Ask your client: Is he prepared for the pain. Most men are not good with pain that is why women have babies. Yet, some men will sit for hours having a tattoo.
- That is a very painful procedure.
- Does he drink alcohol each night after work? Anyone that drinks alcohol on a regular bases feels pain more than someone that does not drink regularly.
- Is he/she taking medication or drugs? Anyone using drugs: - prescribed or recreational must not attend a waxing clinic.

For a man with a plump face. You will need to get him to help with making his facial skin firm. You can ask him to press his lips together and blow air into his closed mouth area. He could also pull his skin towards his ears.

If his hair is what is known as bum fluff or is baby fine, then waxing is a perfectly safe. Otherwise, it is not safe. He could end up with pot holes and scars in his skin.

Men wanting to have their face waxed will need three to six days growth on their face.

EYEBROW WAXING

It is important as a Hair Removal Cosmetologist to be better at your work than a home user that has little or no training.

I have devoted an entire book to eyebrows see My Book devoted to Eyebrows called "Eyebrow Shaping & Coloring to Suit Face Shapes"

Should the eyebrows be the wrong colour or shape to match the clients face shape, hair colour and complexion they will look either, sad, tired, or older than they should.

Calipers are a handy tool to have in your eyebrow shaping toolbox.

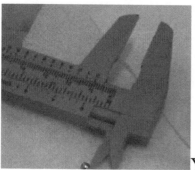

You can use them to check distance between the nose bridge and the arch on each eyebrow.

Therefore, you should: -

- **Study the face.** It is important to give the client a mirror or sit him/her in front of one that you both can look into before you begin. Study his/her face shape. Ask what type of shape he/she wants. If it is his/her first visit to your salon fill in a client card.

- Does he/she just want a tidy up or a reshape to suit her/his face shape?

- **What Type of Eye Treatment Do They Want?** Does your client want a wax treatment? Threading or Plucking? The client may also need her eyebrow hairs tinted if so, do this first.

- Be prepared to offer eyebrow extension.

- **Have Enough Hair.** Eyebrow hair needs to be at least 1/4" long for waxing or plucking. For threading you can remove hair that are barely showing.

- **Decide on the shape of the brows.** Refer to eyebrow shape diagram if you need help deciding on which hairs to take and leave.

- **Pull or pin-back hair.** You want to see the eyebrows clearly, and not get any wax in their hair. Put a disposable cap on.

- **Trim eyebrows if necessary.** Brush their eyebrows straight up, if there are any hairs or longer hairs coming out of their natural shape on top, then you need to trim. Use a fine-tooth eyebrow comb or an eyebrow brush to push eyebrow hair up. Trim what is outside the shape with small scissors (preferably eyebrow scissors).

- **Eyebrow Diagram:** Have several diagrams on a sheet of cardboard laminated to show the client. You can purchase stencils on headbands. They allow you to demonstrate to your client different eyebrow shapes.

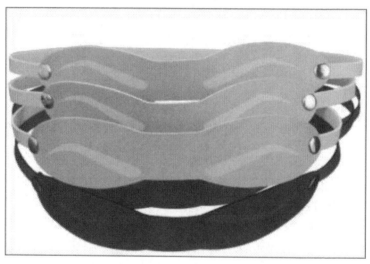

Although diagrams like this assist in communicating with the client before and after photos are your best tool.

- Always take before and after photos.
- Always do a consultation with new clients.
- Always charge more for their first visit unless they just want a quick tidy up.

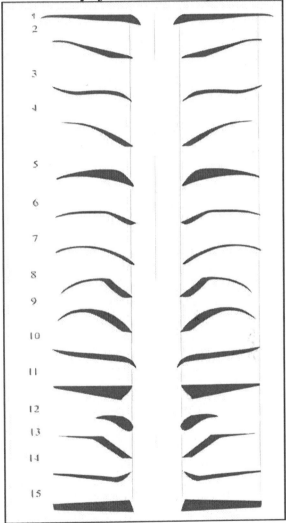

EYEBROW ARCH PLACEMENT

First mark the center of the bridge.

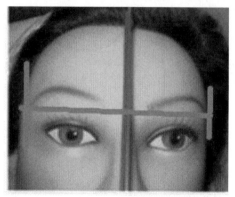

Next the width of their brows.

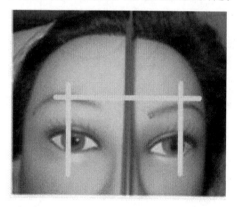

Next, the outside edge of their pupils.

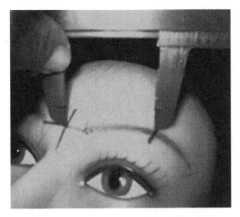

Next the end position of the brow lift. Do so, on both sides of the face. At this point the eyebrow shape, should start to move down

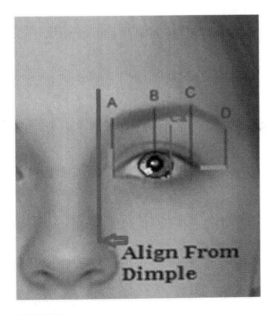

FIGURE 1

Consider these points as well and the type of nose they have. When the client, has a broad nose, start at the dimple. See Figure 2.

Position "A." Will always start in line with either the outer edge of the nose. A wide nose, alignment should start from the dimple in the nose.

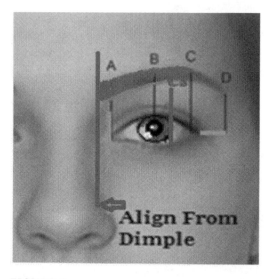

FIGURE 2

Position "B." The eyebrow should have slightly tapered as you reach the "B" mark, which is the center of the eye pupil.

Position "C. " Position "C" is for a peaked type of arch. The peak should be almost at the end of the eyelids outer corner.

Position "Ca." A curved arch should be lined up to start at the end of the pupil. Be sure the client is looking straight ahead.

Position "D." The end of the brow should be a thumb space away from the outer corner of the eyelid or half the width of your nose.

Compare the two alignment photos. Everyone will have a different opinion. In this second photo (Figure 2 above) I have filled in her brow from the dimple alignment, and the inner eye edge "A" plus I gave her a slightly thicker and darker brow. This I believe sends the focus away from her broad nose tip to the center of the nose.

Am I right or am I wrong? This would be an option; you could give a client and have them decide. The first photo (figure 1) with the wider gap between eyebrows, is softer, but the focus is on her nose tip.

With my eyebrows on my right side I follow the nature hair growth. On my left side I add colour to the underside of my peak as my left brow tail sits higher than the tail on my right brow.

Remember there are no two faces that are identical shapes. Therefore, the shaping rules are **not** set in concrete.

To assist a mature face- look younger, you do not always lift the brow, by removing hair from under the brow.

Sometimes you need to add a line with powder shader or cosmetic tattooing to the underside of the brow.

Even if I give you a million photos of eyebrow shapes and ways to shape each or show you those million photos with three different ways to shape each person's eyebrows, there would still be more information you would require.

Learn the basics and use your sixth sense to glamorise a person's face. Practice on family and friends.

Offer your client an eyebrow tidy-up or a full consultation for an eye enhancement treatment.

An older face should have a higher arch then they have had when they were a younger person as it will lift their facial features. Consider a strong center with a lifted tail. If their eyebrows have thinned out you should suggest they have cosmetic tattooing, or eyebrow extensions.

HAIR THREADING TECHNIQUE.

Threading Eyebrows: Photo Compliments of SMH. However, this photo shows the thread being held with both hands.

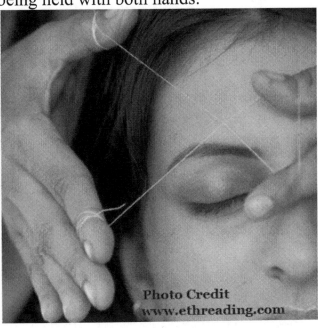

The correct method is to hold the thread with one hand, the other end should be held, with your teeth. That allows for, one hand to be used for holding the skin under the thread tight so you do not gather skin under the thread. It is very easy to tear the skin with this method. I always ask the client to hold their skin as well.

Be sure to powder the eyebrow area for a better grip. Use thick cotton. You can also use string. I prefer string.

If tweezers give your client the willies and waxing sounds cruel or they have very sensitive skin then threading will most definitely be the

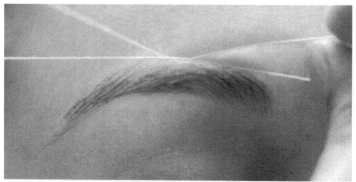

hair removal technique for your client. See what happens when hair is threaded on YouTube videos.

Don't Thread Eyebrows of Mature Skin. Unless, you are very well practiced, in threading art and have an off-sider to assist with holding the skin taut. It is a rolling movement across the skin surface. Then a pull of one end, of the cotton. Therapist roll the skin between the thread and that tears the skin. Yes, you well be rolling the skin with the tread to gather the hair. But at the exact point where the thread crosses, it also gathers soft skin tissue. This causes mature skin to bruise or tear.

PRACTICE THREADING

Cut cotton thread twice the width of the face.

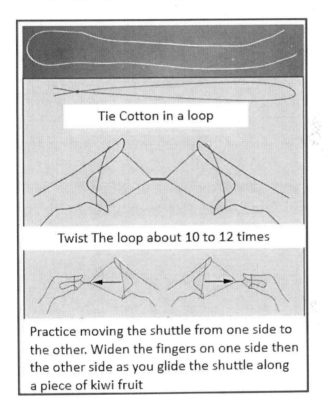

Tie Cotton in a loop

Twist The loop about 10 to 12 times

Practice moving the shuttle from one side to the other. Widen the fingers on one side then the other side as you glide the shuttle along a piece of kiwi fruit

Tie Cotton into a loop

Twist loop about 10 to 12 times your fingers must be inside the loop each end.

Practice moving the shuttle from one side to the other. Widen the fingers on one side then the other side as you glide the shuttle along a piece of kiwi fruit or another type of fruit that is fury.

BASIC FACTS ON THREADING

Eyebrow threading is called khite in Arabic and fatlah in Egyptian, it's a less common method in the West for removing hair at the root, used primarily on facial hair. Rows of stray hairs are pulled out with twists of a cotton thread or thin string.

For a DIY application, watch this, young woman.

https://www.youtube.com/watch?v=eWkrVzhuqrE

In the next YouTube video, the young woman shows and explains shaping as she threads. She has a lovely roll along the skin method as she pulls the hair out. Worth - watching.

https://www.youtube.com/watch?v=KaEWIk9g9UI

THREADING DESCRIPTION:

The practitioner holds one end of the cotton thread in his or her teeth and the other in the left hand. The middle is looped through the index and middle fingers of the right hand. The practitioner then uses the loop to trap a series of unwanted hairs and pull them from the skin. There are also devices made that can hold the thread during the procedure.

For home users the thread is shorter. At home it is impossible to keep the skin firm.

THREADING EYEBROWS ADVANTAGES:

Inexpensive, fast, neat, considered less painful than plucking for many. A good method for eyebrows, and facial hair.

Can be used - to remove hair from any part of the body.

It is a germ-free method when done the right way.

Like plucking, results can last up to two to four weeks. This method is hard to learn but once you learn it, you'll be glad you did.

THREADING EYEBROWS DISADVANTAGES:

Hard to find, a professional practitioner outside large cities. Can be painful and cause itching afterwards. Side effects can include folliculitis, a bacterial infection in the hair follicles, skin reddening or puffiness, and changes in skin pigment.

Not suitable for skin that is maturing.

CLINICAL DATA:

Abdel-Gawar 1997

Chicago Tribune staff reporter Quynh-Giang Tran wrote a nice **article** dated September 9, 2001 "Ancient technique raising-- and shaping-- area eyebrows"

Costs**:**

$20 per treatment for eyebrows; more for larger areas

BACKGROUND FACTS

Marketing terms and tactics:

Historical overview:

The history of threading is not clear, with some claiming it began in Turkey. Threading hair is so basic to women in the Middle East and India that it can be, compared to girls learning to braid each other's hair as children. Traditionally, threading is used on the entire face, including upper lip, chin, eyebrows, sideburns and cheeks. In Chicago, salons performing it can be found in the Indian and Muslim neighbourhoods. Most American cosmetologists are not trained in the procedure and mores the pity. In Australia to-date it is not offered as a module in beauty schools.

GOVERNMENT REGULATION:

Many states require a cosmetologist or aesthetician's license to do hair removal like threading. Putting talcum powder close to the eyes is an art and dangerous when untrained. Threading correctly takes a lot of practice. Check with your local Council as to what their health and safety regulations are pertaining to threading.

BASIC BIKINI WAXING STYLES:

A Basic Bikini wax removes the hair outside the panty line. At the appointment setting time you need to ask, if it is their first bikini wax, or are they, just booking in for a tidy up. Should it be their first time be sure to have a look before quoting on the treatment? Some clients, have very dark think deeply rooted hairs and will require special treatment.

I always warm this type of clients skin first and give them a five-minute tens machine treatment before waxing. Tens machines are a must have, in today's Salons. They are inexpensive and can be a wonderful tool for clients with any kind of aches and pains. A pulse treatment with a Tens machine should be given, to a client as a complimentary treatment prior to bikini waxing.

There are stencils you can purchase for Bikini wax shapes.

BIKINI WAX PROCEEDURE

1. Conduct the meet and greet.
2. Check the client hair type and growth.
3. Fill in Client forms.
4. Clean the area with a pre-wax treatment
5. Apply some gel to the tends machine pads
6. Apply the pads close to the groin but more towards the vagina.
7. Leave on for 5 minutes.
8. Remove and place paper towel over the vagina and groin area
9. Then apply a warm towel
10. Pat dry
11. Apply pre wax oil
12. Apply hot wax not a strip wax in small sections and remove.
13. Press each section with your hand as soon as the wax is pulled off, the section.
14. Apply an astringent.
15. Apply an oil.

Apply a cold cloth and the ice pack.

FULL BIKINI WAX:

Takes the sides of the bikini line deeper than a regular bikini wax, and can also include waxing some hair on top to make a more defined 'triangle' area, or trimming down the hair left shorter.

When to choose full Bikini Wax

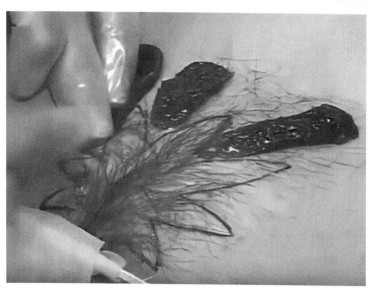

The client still wants to keep hair, but wants more definition than a clean-up. The client may want some shaping and this is when stenciling should be offered at an extra cost. You can use stencils to draw the shape or cut shapes with cardboard and draw around the cardboard. You then wax in small sections. In the above photo the student has not pre-trimmed and most definitely should have.

She has also put wax on a few sections this is not a good practice. Do one section at a time.

FRENCH BIKINI WAX:

Takes all hair off the front (except a small strip) and continues to right before the back of their body. It doesn't take hair off from the back like a Brazilian (see below).

When to Choose a French Bikini Wax

They want the area basically pretty smooth with most hair removed, but do **not** want to take any hair away from behind.

BRAZILIAN BIKINI WAX:

Far too many Therapists, think a Brazilian means all off. It does not. A Brazilian wax takes all hair off the bikini line front, all the way to the back of their posterior (bum). Some folk have unsightly hair growing in the groin and crotch area, these groin hair needs to come off as well.

A small strip or triangle is left in the front and **no** hair is removed from inside the buttock, or the lip of the vagina.

When to choose a Brazilian Wax: The perfect option if they wear a thong bikini, or want to be completely or almost hairless in front and back.

Remember to allow your client to be in control of their bikini wax. You're the technician your client preferences of where and how much hair they want removed or left is to be communicated with them professionally. They can adjust the style to suit their needs and wants. A Young therapist should not perform a Brazilian wax it will offend a client if a teenager is sent into the Beauty Room.

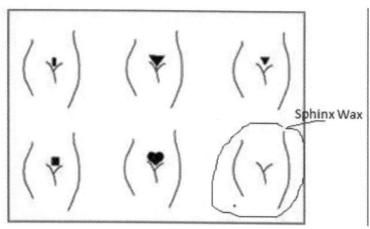

All the shapes except the last one is classed as a Brazilian. A Brazilian wax does not take hair from the lip area of the vaginas opening.

Brazilian bikini waxes have been "all the rage" since the late 90's, but they're certainly not new in the United States.

Brazilian waxing was introduced to New York in 1987 by seven Brazilian-born sisters.

So how does it differ from a regular bikini wax? Mostly, all hair is removed in the front, back and everything in between. Most of the time a "landing strip" is left in the front, but some clients opt for everything removed. Everything removed is called triple x or sphinx wax.

TRIPLE X OR SPHINX

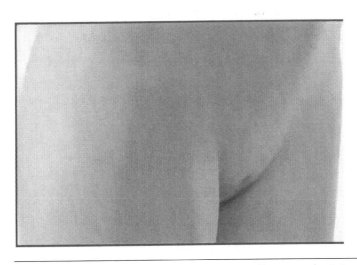

A Triple-X or Sphinx wax includes a full Brazilian but also removes the landing strip and hair from inside the buttock. Be sure to place a tissue inside the vagina to cover the clitoris.

A junior therapist is not allowed to perform a Triple x or Sphinx wax. The triple X and Sphinx waxing requires a separate waxing certificate.

When removing hair from inside the anus there are a few precautions you must follow.

This should only be done in a salon where a warm shower is provided to the client.

The rectum is never fully emptied after passing a motion. Therefore, you must be certain the client is very clean.

- You need to know; they have passed a bowel motion that morning. The motion needed to be a firm one and was not runny.
- While taking a shower they must exfoliate the anus. However, this should have been done a few days ago.
- An anus wax, must be performed straight after the shower while the skin is still warm.
- Be sure the client has washed and dried the area fully.

Face and Body Waxing - Cosmetology

- Have the client positioned like a dog with their bum in the air facing you.
- Sugar or hot wax is best for this treatment.
- Trim long hair.
- After cleaning the anus with astringent, apply talc.
- Wax in small sections.
- Have the client resting on their elbows or chest as they can assist in the pulling of the skin with at least one hand.
- Place a tissue over the clitoris.
- Clients should be on her knees with knees spread apart

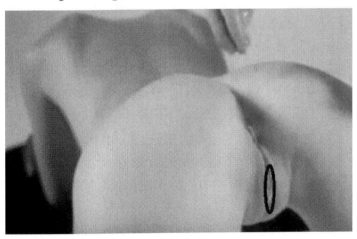

NIPPLE WAXING

Nipple waxing ouch.... A Nipple wax can hurt so the therapist needs to be very careful not to tear the nipple tissue known as **Areola**. If there are just a couple of hairs heat the skin first then remove with the tweezers. If the client has lots of hair use a gentle face hot wax. Position the breast so the nipple lays flat. Have the client help hold the breast firm.

Before you begin you need to have asked the client do, they have or have they had breast cancer or has any family member during the last three generation of blood relatives had breast cancer. If the answer is yes to any of those question, then you should decline the nipple wax session. The client well be well advised to shave her nipples. A discharge could be either a sign of pregnancy or cancer. In both cases the client is not suitable for nipple waxing.

Sometimes you actually need to gentle squeeze the nipple of both male and female clients before a discharge can be noticed.

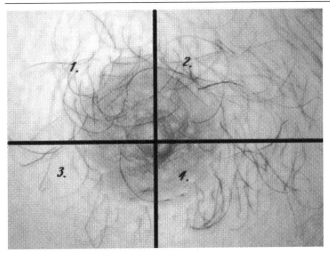

Think of the nipple as four parts and only wax one part at a time. This person nipple hair would require comb over scissors trim first.

1. Clean the nipple with a good cleanser.
2. Check for contra-indications.
3. Tone the skin
4. Trim long hairs but not to short.
5. Apply the pre wax oil or powder.
6. Apply the hot wax.
7. In one section
8. Pull the skin near the nipple very firm

9. Remove the wax in section 1 and press your palm down firmly on the nipple as soon as you pull the wax off. Pressing the newly waxed skin immediately alleviates pain.
10. Continue with the other three sections.
11. Clean the nipple.
12. Apply an ice pack.
13. Apply moisturizer.

UNDER ARM WAXING

1. Clean the area
2. Apply Toner with a cotton wool pad.
3. Apply pre-wax oil or powder.
4. Client hand should be placed under her head.
5. Client needs to assist by pulling her skin towards her chest.
6. Apply a round shaped amount of hot wax
7. Remove wax
8. Apply pressure with the palm of your hand.

Repeat steps 3-6 until you have completely removed all the hair.

7. Apply ice.
8. Wipe dry.

9. Apply Aftercare.

Never wax over the same spot twice as the skin here is very sensitive to heat.

For this reason, chose the pattern of removal wisely.

Long hairs should be trimmed first.

Ask client to pull skin in the opposite direction to the way you will remove the wax is extremely important.

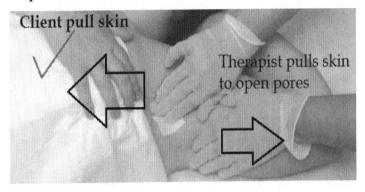

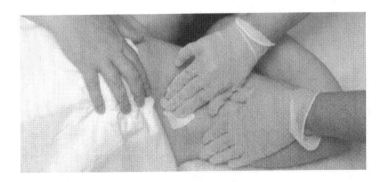

DEEP ARM PIT CHALLENGE.

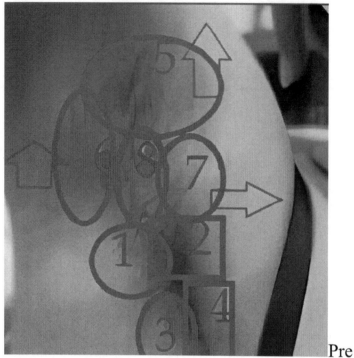

Pre trim long hair. Plan a careful design and wax in small sections.

One section at a time.

CHEST WAXING WOMEN

Depending on how much hair there is and how long the hair is your pattern must be decided before you begin. Always start on the outside edge. This way there will be some hairless skin and some skin with hair. Apply wax in strips, like mowing the lawn. If you do not run down the row the right way, you will have a section of long hair that needs to be waxed but the wax will need to be placed on an area that has already been waxed. With waxing you cannot run more wax over an area that has already been waxed so keep an eye on how you run the wax down your rows. The skin is in a healing mode, and to add more hot wax will create a burn to the skin.

For hair longer than 1.5 cm you will need to pre-trim, using the comb over scissors method or electric clippers with a number 1 comb attached.

CHEST WAXING MEN

Read the above info on chest waxing women.

With scissors over comb start the trim in the center. Electric clippers can be used with the number 1 comb attached.

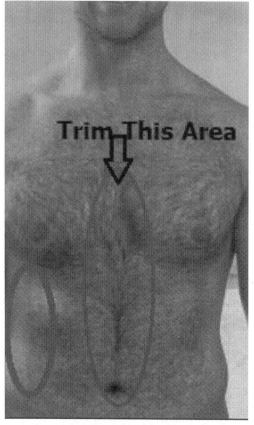

Start wax from the area I have marked in red. The bear patch of skin.

Place a pillow covered in paper towel under the arch in his back This helps to stretch the skin on his stomach.

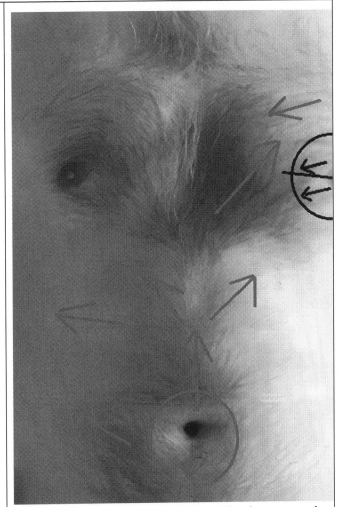

Hair needs to be removed, the way it grows. Pull wax off in opposite direction to the way it flows. In this case there are several directions.

For both men and women, the chest hair grows in several different directions. Therefore, attention to the direction is paramount. Apply the wax in sections in the direction of the growth and remove it in the opposite direction.

BACK WAXING

The back will be waxed with the same rules as for the chest.

LEG WAXING

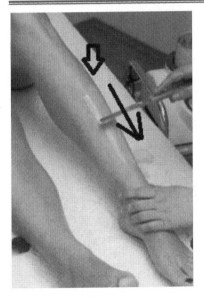

Lower leg wax.

Start with the client lying on her back. Ask her to bend one leg and point her toes.

Wax from below the knee towards the foot unless the hair is growing sideways.

Remove the wax in the opposite direction.

Use the palm of your hand not your finger tips to tighten the skin before pulling off the wax. You must pull in the opposite direction to the movement of the wax removal direction.

Have the client lay on her side with her legs separated. Her knee should be bent. Her toes should be pointed. Now wax the inside of one leg and the outside of the other leg.

When she lays on her stomach have her bring her foot under her leg to tighten the muscles of the leg.

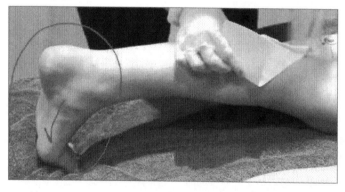

KNEE WAXING

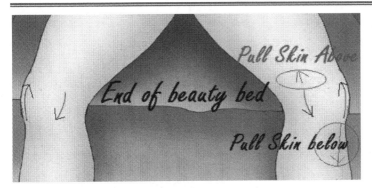

Always wax the knees last after the rest of the legs have been waxed. Have the client sit or lay on the end of the bed with her knees bent over the end of the bed.

Skin lifting causes bruising and is painful. Therefore, you must hold the skin very firmly and pull in the opposite direction on the skin, to the direction the wax is being pulled. Opposite to hair growth direction.

THIGH - UPPER LEG WAX

Bend the clients leg into a figure 4.

Get client to put one hand under the thigh and pull the skin.

This are can bruise very easily

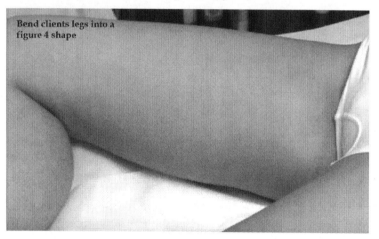

Wax in sections.

Ask the client to pull the skin taut.

Outer Thigh Position

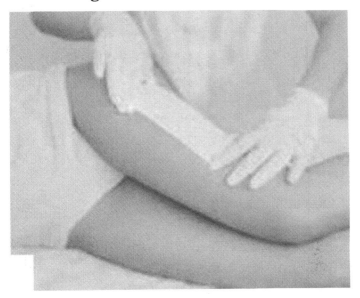

TOES WAXING

Toes can be troublesome. Most people have cold feet even in the summer time. Wax does not stick to cold skin. Toes are also very bonny.

Toe waxing can also be a great add-on for pedicures. It gives the client that little extra pampering so they know their entire foot will be smooth and clean for uninhibited thong/sandal wear and bare feet flashing.

1. Prep toes with your favorite cleanser to remove any lotion or oils from the toes and wipe them dry.

2. Apply a heat bag to each foot.

3. Use Hot wax not strip wax or do sugaring.

4. If toe hair is particularly long, trim with brow scissors, being sure not to trim too short. You want the wax to adhere to the hair not the skin.

5. Bend each toe over your finger.

6. Apply wax to one toe at a time in the direction of the hair growth.

7. At this point, use the "pat and pull" method. Just press for a few seconds and then pull. Continue to do this until the hair is completely removed. The Best method is the "pat and pull" method because rubbing can cause the wax to become imbedded in the cracks of the toe, making it difficult to remove even when you pull the toe taut.

8. After removing hair from all the toes, apply ice and a soothing lotion. finger waxing

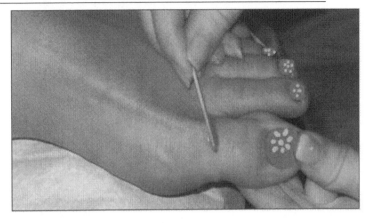

For finger waxing do the same as you would for the toes.

OTHER THINGS TO KNOW

Most wax treatments occur in a private room with a door (although I have heard of some with just a curtain between you and others). A client will be left alone to remove pants and underwear and be asked to lie on a table with clean paper over the towels/sheets. Some clients prefer to be provided, with a paper thong so be sure to enquire if they would like one.

Because a client only needs about a 1.5 cm of hair for the wax to grab onto, it may be best to trim pubic hair to the correct length.
Liberally apply talcum powder to the skin. Talcum powder keeps hot wax from sticking to skin. Or, apply oil depending on the manufactures requirements.
The best wax therapists are fast, which means less discomfort for the client.

Dip a waxing stick into a pot of hot wax and then spread it onto skin and hair in the direction of the hair growth.

For strip wax apply a cloth strip over the still-warm wax, pressing firmly so the cloth, hair and wax adhere to one another. When the wax has cooled, pull the strip off, in the opposite direction of your hair growth, pulling the hairs out by the root.

If using a hot wax, you will remove with your fingers as you do not require a strip of cloth.

Tweeze any stray hairs
Waxing usually starts in the front and moves toward the back. Ask client to assist with holding the skin taut.

Spread soothing lotion over the waxed areas. You should explain what to do in case of bumps, redness, or ingrown hairs.

Tips:

I. Test a small amount of wax on your wrist, before putting on your body part, to make sure the wax is warm, not hot. However, as explained in wax types you should know by the look and consistency of the wax.

II. If you have varicose veins or phlebitis do not wax legs.

III. Read: *Waxing Precautions & Warnings* **for the full list.**

IV. Use After- wax lotion, or aloe-based gel

Note: As an Aromatherapist, I never use baby oil or petroleum jelly on my clients. If they have allergies use Olive Oil. I usually make up a mix of 100 ml Olive Oil with a 4 drops of Rose Geranium 4 drops of Lemon Essential Oil.

Baby Oil and Petroleum Jelly are petroleum chemicals.

TIPS ON GENITAL AREA WAXING:

1. The waxing procedure, can be very painful at first, but frequent visits usually cut down on the pain factor. Suggest taking a couple Pain relief tablets at least 15 minutes (preferably an hour) before your procedure. As for the embarrassment factor -- we like to think getting a Brazilian can't be any more embarrassing than a typical visit to your gynecologist's office.

2. The downside of a Brazilian wax... while it lasts as much as 3 weeks, the hair will grow back and you'll have to do it again.

3. Another downside... hair has to be a certain length before it can be successfully waxed.

4.

5. Waxing can last up to two months depending on hair growth cycle.

PRE-BRAZILIAN WAXING PREP:

TELL YOUR CLIENT

- For women, they need to make an appointment at least a couple days week before or after their period. It is not a good idea to do a Brazilian while they are on their period, and **waxing hurts a lot more during that time anyway.**

- The full moon is a sensitive time for people but do not tell them this just pamper more during this time.

- Shower and lightly exfoliate your entire bikini area at least two days before your appointment using warm, not hot water. On appointment day. Make sure you're extra clean.

- Don't use any lotions in bikini area nor any other area to be waxed.

- You need some growth for the wax to hold onto, but not too long which can make the waxing hurt more than it needs to. Your technician may trim hair down to just the right length at your appointment, or follow the salon's specific instructions for trimming. *There should be a charge for trimming usually $20 or more*

- Take an aspirin 30- 45 minutes before your appointment if you're worried about pain, only if it is safe for you to do so.

If your Salon is near a beach have a big sign in your salon.

Please Shower before arriving for a treatment. We just like you love the beach but we do not want the beach in our salon.

Sand is an absolute menace it gets into everything and some vacuum cleaners do not get every grain of sand. Not only that, you do not want to spend a half hour after a client leaves - cleaning the beauty room.

POST BRAZILIAN WAXING CARE:

Things to say to the client.

- Don't wear tight panties for the next few days.
- Keep hands away from touching freshly waxed skin, as this can encourage irritation or small pimples.
- Don't take a hot bath for the rest of the day.

- No tanning beds, saunas, or steam rooms for the next 2 days.
- Two full days later use a mild exfoliate.
- If you get any ingrown hairs try Tend Skin, a huge favourite for getting rid of pesky in-grown hair.
1. **Have enough hair.** Grow leg hair out to at least 1.5 cm long.

HAIR GROWTH SYSTEM

You may think that this is not important as you only want to get rid of the hair. But this will explain why you have re-growth the next day after shaving, or soon after waxing etc.

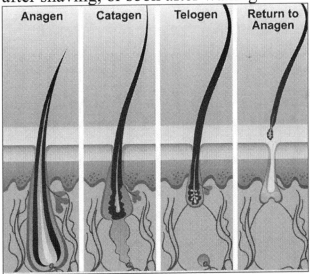

Face and Body Waxing Expectation

1. Anagen onset hair tomorrow will feel like bristles.

2. Exogen hair will be at the skin surface within a few days and feel like bristle and in another few days to a week will feel soft. At this stage your waxed area will start to look a little untidy.

3. Anagen, Catagen, Telogen hair growth takes from 1 to six weeks.

4. The Anagen hairs will be long enough for waxing in 2 to 3 weeks.

Sharing is caring and a smart therapist explains this hair cycle to their client.

It is wise to have a purchased photo of the hair growth cycle in your beauty room.

After cleaning the body wax area - be sure to have the **client confirm** how smooth the waxed area feels.

Next explain the 4 above points. This is called professionalism. It is your job to educate your clients so they know what to expect.

ANAGEN:

The active growing stage - follicle has reformed. The hair bulb is developing surrounding the life-giving dermal papilla, and a new hair forms, growing from the matrix in the bulb.

MITOSIS:

Mitosis is the process of cell division or reproduction, which, after a series of changes within the cell, produces two new identical cells. This occurs in human tissue, including the hair and skin. Groups of similar cells form body tissues, which have specific functions and they may be classified as follows:

Epithelial, connective nerve, muscular and blood.

CATAGEN:

The transitional stage from active to resting. The stops growing and the follicle begins to shrink, or a new hair begins at the base of the follicle as the old hair moves up slowly up the follicle. Here it stays until it falls out, or is pushed out by the new hair.

TELOGEN:

The resting stage - some hair follicles don't undergo the stage as they produce new hair immediately. Hairs may still be loosely inserted in the shallow follicle.

HAIR TYPES

LANUGO:

Hairs found on the foetus – soft and fine, often un-pigmented and no medulla. They are shed after 7 – 8 months of pregnancy and replaced by Vellus hairs except for the hair on the lashes, eyebrows, and scalp; terminal hairs replace these. Some people with alopecia have fine hair with no medulla and need a wax as this fine hair on their scalp will cause itching under the wig. Give these clients a special discount or a 2nd wax session for free.

Have an Aromatherapist make you some merchandizing products to assist with the clients itching.

VELLUS:

Soft, fine, and downy hairs on the body and face, also often un-pigmented. If stimulated, shallow follicles can grow downwards and become a follicle that produces Terminal hairs.

TERMINAL:

Course and longer than Vellus hairs. Most are pigmented – varying greatly in diameter, length, shape, texture and colour. Deep set follicle in the dermis. Terminal hair can be found - bikini, underarm, legs etc.

HIRSUTISM:

A hair growth that is abnormal for that person's sex, e.g., woman's hair growth follows the pattern of a man's hair growth.

HYPERTRICHOSIS:

Is an abnormal growth of excess hair. Usually due to abnormal conditions brought about by injury or disease.

SUPERFLUOUS:

(Excessive hair) Is normal at certain periods in a womens life e.g., during puberty and pregnancy. When hormonal imbalance Vellus hairs can form into Terminal hair and return once imbalance is returned (due to increase in blood supply providing nourishment and encourage growth). Menopause – newly formed hair during menopause is often permanent – can be treated with permanent hair removal, e.g., Electric depilation.

The desire to remove excess or dark hair usually begins in adolescence and seems to continue until the day we die. Whether it is hair on the face, armpits, legs, bikini line, or other body parts, many women AND men are intent upon having the hair on their scalp be the only visible hair on their bodies. With the emphasis on smooth, hairless skin, it is interesting to note that excess hair, especially in women, is still a taboo subject.

There are many options available to remove unwanted hair, but few options to get rid of hair permanently. The different methods of hair removal from the old stand-by, shaving, to the new treatments, lasers and Vaniqa creams need to be discussed, with the client. Each person should choose a method or combination of methods that works best for them depending on cost, time available, skin type, and the desired hair-free area.

HAIR GROWTH

Understanding how hair grows helps us understand how to keep hair from growing. Each hair is contained in a **pilosebaceous unit**, which consists of a hair shaft, hair **follicle**, sebaceous gland, and erector pili muscle. Hair growth and shedding is a continuous cycle through 3 phases. The **anagen** phase is the growth phase, the **catagen** phase is a transitional state, and the **telogen** phase is the resting phase. Hairs spend a variable amount of time in each phase determined by genetics, hormones, and area of the body. Hair in the anagen phase is more susceptible to injury than hair in the telogen phase. All of these factors must be considered when choosing a method of hair removal.

BLEACHING

Bleaching is actually not a hair removal method, but rather a way to make the hair less noticeable. This is especially useful for areas that already have thin but dark and therefore noticeable hair like the arms, face, or neck. Bleaching is performed by applying a chemical to the desired area, which removes the pigment from the hair. Hair bleaching products must be purchased from

Beauty Suppliers. Do Not use hair bleach or house-hold bleaches on your skin. In fact, hair bleach should not be put onto the scalp either. These days when a client goes into a Hairdressing Salon to have her hair bleached, she needs to sign a "Disclaimer" A Hairdresser and Beauty Therapist, can no longer gain insurance for the hair or scalp that has been damaged by bleach. This is why before and after photos help you stay safe. Contact a hairdressing supplier for a quality bleach. It will come with instructions.

How long does facial hair bleaching last?

about 20-25 days

Is face bleaching permanent? The effect of bleaching is temporary and will last for about 20-25 days. The reason is your skin is a dynamic organ which gets affected by sun exposure, hormonal changes, smoking, pollution and even nutrition. Plus it is constantly growing.

CLIENT RELEASE AND INFORMED CONSENT FOR HAIR BLEACHING/LIGHTENING

Students, you need to adjust this form to suit the service you intend to give the client. For waxing clients you may need to add an explanation about hair growth and another section that pertains to aged skin.

Face and Body Waxing - Cosmetology

Clients Name _____
Suburb _____
Date Of Birth _____ Mobile _____
Home or Office Phone _____

1. I understand that the bleaching and/or lightening process will produce different results in different hair types. _____ (Initial)

2. 2. I understand that if I have boxed colour, dark colour, fashion colour or naturally dark hair colour, it may take multiple sessions to achieve the desired lightness of my hair. _____ (Initial)

3. 3. I understand that because everyone's hair is different, my hair may not look exactly like any picture that I have shown my hairstylist. _____ (Initial)

4. 4. I have been honest with my stylist about the colour and chemical history of my hair. I understand that if I have intentionally or unintentionally failed to disclose any information regarding the colour and/or chemical service history of my hair, that the results of my hair bleaching and/or lightening may be unpredictable and that I cannot hold __ (name of salon)

Face and Body Waxing - Cosmetology

_____responsible for the outcomes, and that I am responsible for paying for the cost of the service in full regardless of the outcomes. _____ (Initial) 5. I understand that the blonding process will alter the condition (meaning texture, elasticity, and porosity) of my hair. _____ (Initial

5.) 6. My stylist, _____ has explained to me that bleaching and/or lightening my hair may result in damage and/or breakage of my hair. _____ (Initial) 7. I have been informed that the cost of my service today (date of service) will be $ _____ and I agree to pay this full cost for today's service. _____ (Initial) 8. I understand that it may not be possible to change my hair colour back to its original colour after bleaching and/or lightening my hair. _____ (Initial) 9. I understand that if I choose to change my hair back to its original colour after bleaching and/or lightening my hair, I will be responsible for the cost of that service. _____ (Initial) 10. I release__ (name of salon) _____ from any legal liabilities resulting in bleaching and/or

lightening my hair. _____ (Initial) By signing my name, I agree to the terms and conditions above and to the service being performed.

6. Signature Date Parent or Guardian if under 18: _____

7. Signature Date_____

HAIR REMOVAL - SHAVING

Shaving is the most temporary method of hair removal because it merely cuts the hair off at the skin surface. Shaving does not make the hair shaft thicker, darker, or grow faster or slower.

However, the short hair shaft may be more noticeable as it grows out because it has a blunt tip instead of the normal tapered tip. Shaving should be done after applying some type of moisturizer to the skin to help the razor glide over the skin, not cut or scrape it. Common moisturizers include water, shaving cream, hair conditioner, or body wash.

PHYSICAL HAIR REMOVAL

Physically pulling the hair out of the follicle is a

common and fairly inexpensive, method of hair removal. None of these methods change the color, texture, or density of the hair. The hair takes longer to grow back because it must grow to the surface of the skin before it is noticed. Because hair grows at different rates, some of the hair that has been physically removed may take more time to grow back in. Repeatedly pulling hair out of the follicle may damage the follicle enough over time to keep it from producing more hair.

PHYSICAL HAIR REMOVAL - PLUCKING

Plucking hair with tweezers is an effective way to remove hair but can be very time consuming. The hair shaft must be long enough to grasp with tweezers.

PHYSICAL HAIR REMOVAL - WAXING

Waxing is an effective method of removing large amounts of hair at one time. In this method wax is warmed to allow it to be spread easily over the skin in the direction of hair growth. The hair becomes embedded in the wax, which cools and firms up grasping the hair. The wax is then quickly pulled off in the opposite direction of the hair growth, pulling the hairs out of the follicles. Cold waxes are available usually attached to strips, which are patted onto the skin. Wax that is still left on the skin must be peeled or scratched off. Caution must be used when heating wax so as not to burn the skin.

AIR BORNE DISEASES

An airborne disease is any disease that is caused by pathogens and transmitted through the air. Such diseases include many that are of considerable importance both in human and veterinary medicine. The relevant pathogens may be viruses, bacteria, or fungi, and they may be spread through:
- coughing,
- sneezing,
- raising of dust,
- spraying of liquids.

or similar activities likely to generate aerosol particles or droplets.

Strictly speaking airborne diseases do not include conditions caused simply by air pollution such as dusts and poisons, though their study and prevention are related.

Airborne pathogens or allergens often cause inflammation in the nose, throat, sinuses, and the lungs. This is caused by the inhalation of these pathogens that affect a person's respiratory system or even the rest of the body. Sinus congestion, coughing and sore throats are examples of inflammation of the upper respiratory air way due to these airborne agents. Air pollution plays a significant role in airborne diseases which is linked to asthma. Pollutants are said to influence lung function by increasing air way inflammation.[1]

Many common infections can spread by airborne transmission at least in some cases, including: Anthrax (inhalational),
- Chickenpox,
- Influenza,
- Measles,
- Smallpox,
- Cryptococcosis,
- Tuberculosis.

An airborne disease can be caused by exposure to a source: an infected patient or animal, by being transferred from the infected person or animal's mouth, nose, cut, wound, or needle puncture. People receive the disease through a portal of entry: mouth, nose, cut, or needle puncture.

QUIZ YOURSELF

Q11 Bleaching fill in the blanks

Bleaching is actually not a _____ removal method, but rather a way to make the hair less _____. This is especially useful _____ but dark and therefore noticeable hair like the arms, face, or neck. Bleaching is performed by applying a chemical to the desired area, which _____ from the hair.

Q12 Hair Removal with Shaving

Shaving is the most _____ method of hair removal because it merely _____ hair off at the skin surface. Shaving does not make the hair shaft _____, darker, or grow faster or slower. However, the short hair shaft may be more noticeable as it grows out because it has a _____ instead of the normal tapered tip. Shaving should be done after applying some type of moisturizer to the skin to help the razor glide over the skin, not cut or scrape it. Common moisturizers include water, shaving cream, hair conditioner, or body wash.

Q13 Physical Hair Removal

Physically pulling the hair out of the follicle is a common and fairly inexpensive method of hair removal. None of these methods changes the color, texture, or density of the hair. The hair takes _____ to grow back because it must grow to _____ of the skin before it is

Face and Body Waxing - Cosmetology

noticed. Because hair grows _____, some of the hair that has been physically removed may take more time to grow back in. Repeatedly pulling hair out of the follicle may damage the follicle enough over time to keep it from producing more hair.

Q14   Physical Hair Removal – Plucking.

Plucking hair with tweezers is an effective way to remove hair but can be ---------------------- consuming. The hair shaft must be long enough to grasp with tweezers.

Q15   Physical Hair Removal – Waxing

Waxing is an effective method of removing large amounts of hair at one time. In this method wax is warmed to allow it to be _____ over the skin in the direction of hair growth. The hair becomes _____ in the wax, which cools and firms up grasping the hair. The wax is then quickly pulled off in the opposite direction of the hair growth, pulling the hairs out of the follicles. _____ waxes are available usually attached to strips, which are _____ onto the skin. Wax that is still left on the skin must be peeled or scratched off. Caution must be used when heating wax so as not to _____ the skin.

ABOUT DO'S AND DON'TS

Firstly, let me say if you are a therapist that offers waxing, this list of Do's and Don'ts & Warnings, should be on your clients' disclaimer form. They should sign before having a wax done.

Do's and Don'ts is always the most important section to read in any training manual. It takes all the learning pages and reduces all you need to know into a few lines or pages. The trouble is that if you don't know your procedures before you read this section it does not have the impact it should have.

However, I loved reading the "One Minute Manager" and found it very helpful in my time management skills. Of cause, I read it after I had already made lots of time management mistakes.

Those of you that are always reading to improve your skills will know exactly what I mean.

My intention here with my do's and don'ts section is to change that equation by adding photos to my do's and don'ts section here and videos to YouTube. I am hoping this helps the beginners to waxing - learn the best methods a lot faster.

DO'S AND DON'TS

WAXING PRECAUTIONS & WARNINGS

Face and Body Waxing - Cosmetology

Be cautioned that during pregnancy, taking birth control, hormone replacement or antibiotics. During these times your skin will be more sensitive to waxing, so it is best to have a patch test (like a small area on your arm) and see how your skin reacts during the next 24 hours before getting an entire eyebrow or leg wax.

Smokers or those with Rosaceae have delicate capillaries and waxing can irritate weak or broken blood vessels. Therefore, they should stay away from waxing on the fac.

Taking blood thinners, if you have diabetes, phlebitis or want post- cancer hair growth in side-burn area removed. These all relate to medical conditions, so first get your doctor's approval before waxing.

Salicylic acid, alpha-hydroxy acid, white willow bark, white willow bark extract and enzymes all strip cells from the skin. It is all too much exfoliation of the skin when combined with waxing, and could make skin red, bleed or

even turn scabby. If the alpha-hydroxy is over 8% then you may have to wait months before safely getting waxed.

Caffeine or alcohol are stimulants in your system and can cause skin to be extra sensitive to waxing, meaning you could become redder or inflamed than usual. Give yourself a couple hours after drinking coffee or alcohol before having a wax treatment.

Do not offer clients to be waxed a cup of coffee, tea, or alcohol.

WHEN NOT TO GET WAXED:

You are currently taking Accutane, or have stopped taking it less than a year ago.

You're taking any prescription acne medication.

You have lupus or AIDS.

You are in cancer therapy getting chemotherapy or radiation.

You have been in direct sunlight for a long period of time or tanning bed within the last 24 hours.

Anywhere on the body that you are using Retin-A

Irritated, inflamed, cut, or sunburned skin.

Any area that has a rash, recent scar tissue, a skin graft, pimples, cold sores, moles, or warts. Anywhere you're having Dermabrasion services or have gotten them in the past three months.

WAXING AFTER CANCER TREATMENT

It is important to be cautious when proceeding with hair-removal techniques such as waxing after cancer treatments, the body is very sore from cancer treatments, or your skin is experiencing some negative effects from the chemotherapy or radiation, it may be best to skip procedures that increase sensitivity such as waxing. Avoid cuts and scrapes that can lead to infection, and wear gloves when providing treatment.

WHEN GOLDEN RULES DON'T WORK.

For someone with a broad nose that would mean that the above-mentioned method {under eyebrow shaping} the line would meet in the center of the bridge.

So, when the nose is broad at the tip, we have to make adjustments as you see here in this photo. We imagine there is a line from the center of the nostrils passing by the inner eye corner and that is where the eyebrow bow should begin.

However, with this young woman even a line from the center of the nostril and touching the inside of the eye point would not work. So, you see there cannot be a Golden rule where people are concerned. It is always best to study the face and ask the client what look she would like. Clients most of the time have a sixth sense that works better than our professionalism.

~~~ *** ~~~

DO'S AND DON'TS PHOTO PAGES

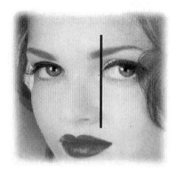

With eyebrow mapping before waxing - we are told to place the stick line at the edge of the nose and line it up with the inside of the eye. In most situations this would be a **"DO"**

However, If the nose is broad at the tip this would be a **"Don't."**

Don't Apply all the wax on the top and bottom of both eyebrows at once.

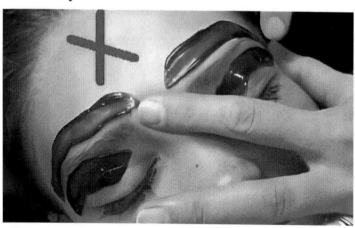

Do map the eyebrows first and have the client approve the shape.

Do brush the eyebrow hairs and trim long hairs Always trim long hair on the face and body. Pulling wax off long hair causes pain and may snap leaving short stumps of hair.

Do follow manufacturers instructions and the product they recommend.

Do Apply the wax on skin in small section.

Do remove each section of wax - before applying the next section of wax.

Do press the was into the skin.

Face and Body Waxing - Cosmetology

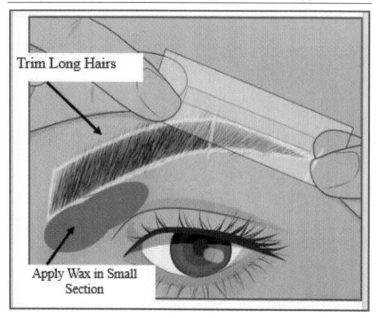

DO: - Always gently pull the skin tight so no wrinkles nor loose skin are present as you place the wax on the skin. Hold for a moment to allow the wax to set before releasing the tension.

Don't use finger tips to push wax into the skin.

Do. When removing strip wax:-.

Face and Body Waxing - Cosmetology

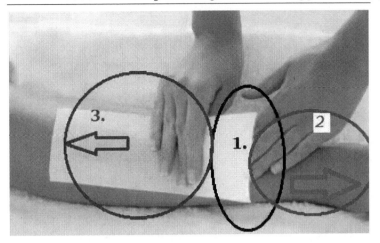

1. Leave a tail of cloth that is not pressed onto the wax. This tail is where you hold the cloth to avoid getting wax on your hands, as you remove the wax.

2 Do rub the strip of cloth into the wax with a firm closed hand. You need to rub back and forward to cause friction. This will push the wax into the skin.

Face and Body Waxing - Cosmetology

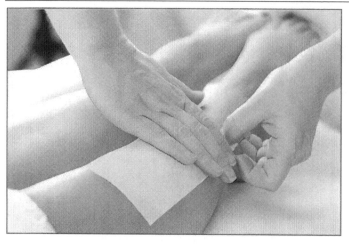

3. After the friction rub - place the palm of your hand at the point near the cloth tip and pull the skin tight in the oposit direction to the way you are going to remove the wax.

4. Pull the hair off in the oposite direction to the hair growth. As you remove the wax with the cloth strip say parrelle to the skink do not pull up towards the ceiling.

Don't Pull the wax strip off if you have not applied friction to the strip. It is plainly obvious that this therapist has not placed her palm on the strip and rubbed the strip enough. The cloth is barely touching the skin. If you do not apply friction to the strip, it will rip the hair off and not pull the hair root out. Also, there is not enough strip left to remove the wax in one full swing.

Face and Body Waxing - Cosmetology

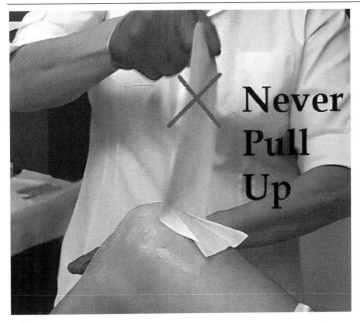

Don't pull the cloth strip up.

Do hold the skin at the base of the pull.

Do move both your body and arm parallel to the skin as you remove the wax. It is a swing movement.

Don't use strip wax for the under arms.

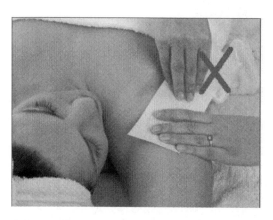

Don't Use Strip wax on under arms

Note -Pressing fingers into warm skin can cause bruising an hour or so after the wax has been completed.

Do Use **Hot Wax** for underarms and on the face. **Not** strip wax.

Her **Do** is- she is using the balls of her fingers to press the wax into the skin.

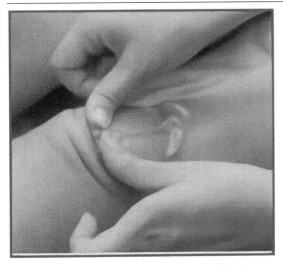

However, she has the clients leg flat on the bed. That is a **Don't.**

Knees up will help stretch the skin and keep it form.

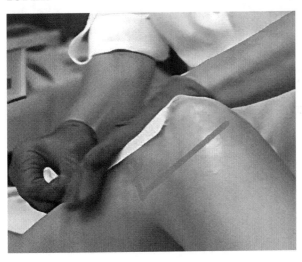

Do: Knees are bent and up for waxing knees. sitting on the end of the bed works best as explained above.

Do - have legs bent when removing wax. Both strip and hot wax are ok for leg waxing.

Do trim long hairs before you wax.

Do This is a perfect way to remove the strip. She is pulling the strip off parallel to the skin. If you pull up and of- the hairs break but if you pull along the skin and off the hairs are more inclined to be removed from the follicle.

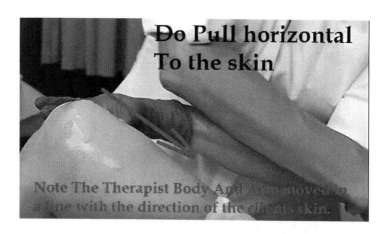

Do Pull horizontal To the skin

Note The Therapist Body And Arm moves in a line with the direction of the client's skin.

The next photo the hand is in the wrong position and should be flat. When you use the tips of your fingers you could leave bruises. I have added arrows and a hand diagram to the photo to hopefully give you an idea on how the hand should be placed. Not the below arrow is indicating the skin pull is in the opposite direction to the wax being pulled off.

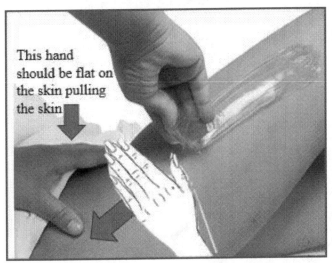

Do- have legs bent when removing wax.

Never pull wax up and off.

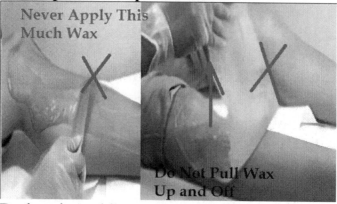

Both strip and hot wax are ok for leg waxing.

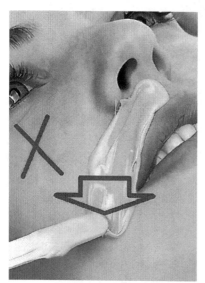

- **Never use this much wax.**
- **Never apply a lip or eyebrow wax in one continuous strip.**
-

Face and Body Waxing - Cosmetology

- Never ever, dip a wax stick into the pot twice.
- Never ever use a roller type wax on more than one client.
- Never ever use roller style wax on the face nor on the arm pit.
- Keep your salon spotlessly clean.
- Sterilize all equipment.
- Use a single use item when possible.
- Always apply wax in small sections this allows you to pull back close to the skin. As you paddle the wax onto the skin do so meticulously with pressure so the wax oozes into the skin pores.

CLIENTS DO & DON'T HAND OUT

The clients hand out should include do and don't list. Make one to give your clients. Try to improve on this information.

Do.

1. Make sure your skin is not inflamed, irritated, cut, infected, sunburn or too dry.

2. Never come to the salon straight from a swim in the river or the ocean.

3. Exfoliate at least 2 to 3 days before your session to remove dead skin. Not the same day of your wax session.

4. Moisturize your skin daily, but do not apply moisturizer on waxing day as it interferes with the wax.

5. A quality night cream or oil should be applied after your evening skincare routine.

6. For anus, triple x, and sphinx waxing you need to have had a good bowel movement one hour before the wax session. Be very clean in that area. Bowels seldom empty completely, please sit on the toilet for an extended time. Our sincere thanks.

Don't...

A. **Do Not -** Apply moisturizer to your face on waxing day.

B. **Do Not -** Exfoliate on waxing day as this makes your skin sensitive and could cause inflammation.

C. **Do Not -** Exercise one hour before your facial waxing.

ADVICE FOR THE BEAUTY THERAPY INDUSTRY

The following information has been developed to assist the beauty therapy industry with questions relating to skin penetration. This information is to be read in conjunction with the Code of Practice for Skin Penetration Procedures (PDF 324KB).

Health inspections of beauty salons

It is the responsibility of the local government environmental health officer to inspect the premises to ensure the owner and employees are complying with the Code of Practice for Skin Penetration Procedures (the Code).

The owner of an establishment who does not comply with the Code is committing an offence, and may face penalties under the Health (Skin Penetration Procedures) Regulations 1998 (external site).

Read more about skin penetration laws and age limits. Most health departments call it "Personal Appearance Services"

Disposal of sharps and contaminated waste. Used wax is considered contaminated material.

It is important to contact your local government environmental health officer to discuss the disposal of contaminated wastes and sharps in your local area.

Visit the Western Australia Local Government Authority (external site) for a list of local government contact details. Beauty therapy regulations are similar worldwide as are the training regulations.

HEALTH RISKS ASSOCIATED WITH BEAUTY THERAPIES

There are a number of health risks associated with the beauty therapy industry.

These include:

Viral infections (for example hepatitis B, hepatitis C, HIV/AIDS) bacterial infections (for example Staphylococcus aureus and Staphylococcus epidermidis) Fungal infections (for example Candida albicans). excessive bleeding, scarring, exposure to toxic chemicals or dyes, allergies.

Terms explained

Critical procedure – this is a procedure where instruments enter or penetrate the skin, for example acupuncture needles, lances, waxing tools, etc.

Semi-critical procedure – this is a procedure where instruments are likely to come into contact with mucosa or blood, but do not penetrate the skin. Such instruments include tweezers, emery boards, cuticle scissors, etc.

Reducing risks associated with beauty therapies
Waxing

Reuse of depilatory wax (is semi-critical procedure)

Body hair can accumulate micro-organisms on the skin. Removing body hair with wax also removes these micro-organisms and contaminates the wax in the process.

Melting down the used wax does not destroy these micro-organisms and reusing this wax could lead to the transmission of diseases such as HIV/AIDS.

It is also important to remember that tiny amounts of blood may also be extracted from small scabs or hair follicles during the waxing process, not all of which will be visible.

All wax must be single use only and disposed of after each use on a client.

Separating unused wax and used wax (semi-critical procedure)

It is important to separate unused wax from wax to be used on a client. This will prevent cross contamination of micro-organisms to the unused wax stock.

To achieve this, all wax should be poured or removed from stock using a new clean spatula or ladle and placed into a clean container prior to each client treatment. If more wax is needed use a new spatula.

If a ladle is being used to remove wax from stock, you do not necessarily need a new ladle each time, provided the ladle does not come into contact with any material that is in use on the client.

Disposable spatulas and containers should be discarded appropriately after use. Wooden spatulas used to apply strip wax should only be used on 1 client and then disposed of. If metal spatulas are used, they must be cleaned and disinfected between clients. You must not put the spatula on the skin to apply the wax, then put back into the wax pot to gather more wax.

Any reusable containers should be cleaned and disinfected between clients.

Roll-on wax (semi-critical procedure)

There are a number of roll-on wax products, on the market where wax is stored in a container and then rolled onto the skin with roller heads.

The wax that is rolled onto the skin may re-circulate back into the container and can contaminate unused wax.

Therefore, once this product is used on one client, the wax in the container must be thermally disinfected before it can be used on a second client (unless the product manufacturer can prove to the Department of Health that the wax in the container will not be contaminated).

The roller head and the container must also be cleaned and disinfected after each use to remove any used wax residue and other micro-organisms.

Advice for clients after waxing

Therapists may wish to advise their clients that after waxing the pores in the skin can remain open for up to 48 hours, making skin more sensitive to ultraviolet light. A cold shower or cold compress help close pores more quickly.

It is recommended therapists advise clients not to sunbathe or to have a solarium treatment for at least 48 hours after being waxed.

Electrolysis (critical procedure)

Electrolysis hair removal involves using a needle to penetrate the skin surrounding a hair follicle. This could result in the contamination of the needles with small amounts of blood and bodily fluids.

The transmission of blood borne infections then becomes possible.

Only single use electrolysis needles are permitted for use in for electrolysis treatments.

Sterile needles must be inserted into the electrolysis equipment at the start of a treatment. The same needle can be used for removing multiple hairs necessary from one client during a single session.

Used needles must be disposed of into a sharps container upon completion of the procedure.

The needle used for one client cannot be stored and then reused for the same client at future electrolysis sessions. A new sterile needle must be used for every treatment.

It is essential that the operator wears clean gloves and has clean hands before and after every treatment session.

Lancing skin (critical procedure)

Lancing of the skin involves treatments such as the removal of blackheads, pimples, and ingrown hairs, by penetrating the skin using a sharp instrument called a lance.

Sterile single use equipment must be used for this process.

Tweezing (semi-critical procedure)
Tweezers should be rinsed off with warm water, then immersed in detergent and water and scrubbed under

water with a clean brush after they have been used on a client.

Where tweezers become contaminated with blood or body fluids they should be cleaned and disinfected between clients in accordance with the Code of Practice for Skin Penetration Procedures.

Nails

Clients with visible nail or skin infections should be referred to a health professional before having a manicure or pedicure.

Pedicures (semi-critical procedure)

During a pedicure treatment it is possible to contract a fungal, bacterial, or viral infection from dirty nail care tools and equipment.

Equipment used for rasping (scraping) corns and calluses on feet should be cleaned and disinfected after each client in accordance with the Code.

It is recommended by the Department of Health that single-use disposable files are used for each client and discarded afterwards. Other non-disposable files and instruments must be cleaned and disinfected in accordance with the Code.

There have been cases of bacterial infections associated with whirlpool foot spas that were not sufficiently cleaned and disinfected on a regular basis.

If you use foot spas in the salon they need to be drained, cleaned, and disinfected after each client. The intake

filter should also be removed, cleaned, and soaked in disinfectant every week.
Note: Clients' feet should be washed prior to a pedicure.

Manicuring (semi-critical procedure)
Fungal, viral, and bacterial infections can be easily spread during manicure treatments. It very easy to cut a client's skin when cutting cuticles or to break the skin if you file too deeply.

To avoid the transmission of infections, it is recommended that all instruments are single use and disposed of immediately after use, or suitably cleaned and disinfected in accordance with the Code.
Any manicure instrument that may have been contaminated with blood or other bodily fluids must be cleaned and disinfected.
Note: Clients should wash their hands prior to a manicure.

Cosmetic tattooing (critical procedure)
Cosmetic tattooing processes involve the same processes as a standard tattooing procedure.
Cosmetic tattooing can also be referred to as:
- micro-pigmentation
- pigment implants
- semi-permanent creations
- permanent makeup, or derma-pigmentation.

Cosmetic tattooing must be performed in accordance with the Code, particularly in relation to sterilizing appliances.

The needle chamber from the permanent cosmetic machines should be detachable so it can be cleaned and sterilized.

Note: There are serious penalties for tattooing a minor in any way. Read more about the age limits for skin penetration procedures.

Creams, powders, or ointments
The most effective way to dispense ointments is by using self-dispensing pump packs. This prevents cross contamination of the ointment.

When refilling pump pack containers, the self-dispensing pump should be cleaned before refilling the container.
To avoid cross-contamination, any products contained in a tub, such as makeup, powders, or creams, should be removed from the container by using a clean single use applicator.

The same applicator should not be used on another client or dipped back into the original container. After removing the applicator from the container, any extra cream or ointment should be disposed of and not returned to the original container.

ULTRAVIOLET LIGHT CABINETS

Ultraviolet (UV) cabinets do not sterilize equipment.

UV light will not penetrate all surfaces of exposed appliances and some viruses, including HIV, can still survive.
Microwave ovens, pressure cookers, incubators, boiling water units, ultrasonic cleaners and other similar appliances are not sterilizing machines.

Similarly, wiping equipment and appliances will not sterilize the item.
More information
Contact your local government environmental health officer.
Phone the Environmental Health Directorate on 61 29388 4999.
Read the Code of Practice for Skin Penetration Procedures (PDF 324KB).
For information on occupational health and safety visit WorkSafe Western Australia (external site) or phone 1300 307 877.

There is a department of Health In every state and country. Now that the International Standards are written and complete, all countries within the international treaties have the same Code of Practice and Training Standards.

AUTOCLAVES

Did you know if you cannot afford an Autoclave for your salon your local Dentist or Hospital will sterilize your tools for a very low cost and they have a daily pickup service from your local doctors surgery? You need to scrub, bag, and tag the tools and record your scrub details and send your scrub book to the Hospital so they can date and sign the sterilizing process.

Face and Body Waxing - Cosmetology

CLIENT HISTORY CARD

A well set out client history card/form can be your saving grace.

Client History					
Full Name				DOB	
Address				P Code/Zip	
Home Phone		Wk Ph:		Mobile	
Lifestyle e.g. Sport, frequency of					
General H	Excellent	Good	Poor	High Blood Pressure	
				Low Blood Pressure	
Explain If F				Pulse Rate	
List Medics For ailmen		Allergies		Skin Type	
				Combination	
				Dehydrated	
				Oily	
				Acne	
				Normal	
				Rosacea	
				Blisters	
How many glasses of alcohol to day				Prone 2Cold Sores	
How many glasses of alcohol last night				Eczema	
What social drugs are you on				Eyes Water	
Carbuncles				Psoriasis	
Arthritis				Celulitus	
Are you Diabetic				Dermatitus	
Kidney issues					

As well as their personal details such as name address phone and a copy of photo Id you need to know certain things about them and they must sign and date the form to imply all they have said is correct.

Face and Body Waxing - Cosmetology

Things you need on this form.

Their skin and hair type. Colour and condition

Is their skin dehydrated, combination of oily, and dry, normal? Do they have acne. Where are their ingrown hairs and what condition are they in. If you or your junior fill in the clients form for them, the client must sign that all is correct and initial the answers.

Skin Type	Answers	Client Initials
Combination		
Dehydrated		
Oily		
Acne		
Normal		
Rosacea		
Ingrown Hairs		
Blisters		
Prone 2 Cold Sores		
Eczema		
Eyes Watery		
Psoriasis		
Cellulitis		
Finger Nail Condition		
Toe Nail Condition		

General health conditions Good Fair Excellent

Do you suffer or have?
Carbuncles
Psoriasis
Arthritis
Cellulitis
Are you Diabetic?
Kidney Issues
Liver issues
Epilepsy
Schizophrenia
Depression levels
HIV
Aides
Bruises & position
Have you been in contact with People with an airborne disease in last 20 days, Measles, Mumps Chickenpox, SARs, Covid19,
Are you pregnant or breast feeding?
Explain Ailment e.g., Torn ligament, blood issues, Rosacea.
Basal cell carcinoma
Squamous cell carcinoma
Melanoma
Lupus
Warts
Impetigo
Hives

Face and Body Waxing - Cosmetology

Ring Worms
How many glasses of alcohol di you have last night?
When did you last take recreational drugs
What did you take. Date ___ Time ___

Nail condition of toes and fingers

Hair colour and type Fine Strong Normal

When an abusive husband comes in it is usually because his wife has told him an untruth. Explain to him he is to deal with his concerns with his wife. His wife is our client and under client confidentiality you cannot discuss her service with him.

Complaints are rare when you are a professional However, they do happen from time to time.

Always take before and after photo

Always have the client feel their wax and confirm it is smooth.

All the answers are correct and true

Sign_____ Date ____

Today I had a _____

by Therapist name goes here _____

Face and Body Waxing - Cosmetology

My wax is smooth with no broken hairs

Sign_____ Date _____

At the end of the salon form always have them state they are happy with the work, name the work.

Take before and after photos and keep with the clients' folder. Always charge for the consolation. Filling in forms is time consuming. Time is money. Always ask client their email address and have them fill in as much of the form as possible. Give them the option to sign a waiver form if they are just coming for a one-off lip or eyebrow wax. If they are not a local, they may not want a consultation.

Things can go wrong therefore - you as a therapist need to protect yourself.

OTHER BOOKS BY ROBYNA SMITH-KEYS

HEALING AND TRAINING MANUALS

Ba Ha Ha Happy!
Foolproof Aromatherapy
The Antique Healer
Dog Care & DIY Organic Medications
Organic Cancer Cure. Note: this cancer book is free. You will find it at all major book sales. But try smashwords.com
Positive Spiritual Affirmations.
Colours That Heal.

TRAINING MANUAL - BEAUTY SCHOOLS

Body Piercing Basics.
Anatomy for Body Piercers.
Eyebrow Shaping & Colouring to Suit Face Shapes.
Eyelash Extensions Grafting Lashes Training Manual.
Face and Body Waxing-Cosmetology.
Cosmetic Tattoo Permanent Makeup Micro-pigmentation.
An Angel for Cosmetic Tattooists
Hair Extensions Training Manual

Supernatural: -

Spell Folklore
Tarot Scrolls 0-22

Children's Books: -
Romeo and Juliette Keep Mark Antony
Mark Antony Marries Lizzy and has Puppies.

~ ** ~

Other books at Beauty School Books by Robyn Ji Smith
site. www.beautyschoolbooks.com.au
Facebook is
 https://www.facebook.com/groups/FolkloreHealings
and
https://www.facebook.com/AromatherapyAndBeautySchoolBooks

- Alluring Study of Aromatherapy For Healers & Perfumers
- D I Y Signature Perfume Creating
- Learn Perfume Creating with Natures Gifts- Subtitle: Organic & Synthetic
- Got It
- DIY Chakra Balancing
- Reiki and Chakra Balancing
- Learn Reiki Energy Healing
- Design & Perform Cosmetic Tattooing Micropigmentation.
- Diaries on Mindfulness and Gratitude.

YOU MAY CONTACT THE AUTHOR AT

Facebook:

http:// www.facebook.com/groups/FolkloreHealings

Twitter: http://www.twitter.com/@AuthorRobyna

Email:

mailto:beautyschoolbooks@gmail.com

I am happy to answer your question via my Facebook group. Never be shy. **Life is about** helping each other. We create a better life - when we are willing to help others without a cost.

Bye for now

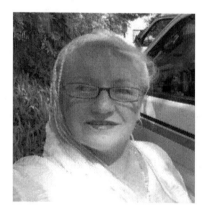

Happy Learning

Robyna XXX

Made in the USA
Middletown, DE
02 December 2024

65939743R00095